# A NEW WARNING SIGN

Plain old cholesterol—the bogeyman red flag of coronary heart disease—may be less of a problem than most people and their doctors realize. The fundamental cause of cardiovascular diseases may be related to homocysteine, a substance produced by the body when the intake of specific vitamins is low. What can you do about it? This health guide explains how the B-complex vitamins—particularly folic acid, vitamins B6 and B12, and choline—neutralize dangerous homocysteine and reduce the risk of disease.

# ABOUT THE AUTHORS

**Jack Challem** is a well-known health writer who has been reporting advances in vitamin and mineral research since 1974. He is the coauthor of *The Natural Health Guide to Beating the Supergerms* (Pocket Books/Simon & Schuster, 1997). His other books include *What Herbs Are All About* (Keats, 1981), *Getting the Most Out of Your Vitamins and Minerals* (Keats, 1993), and *The Health Benefits of Soy* (Keats, 1996).

Challem writes and publishes *The Nutrition Reporter*™ newsletter and is a contributing editor to *Let's Live, Natural Health,* and *Nutrition Science News* magazines. He also writes for *Health Naturally* (Canada), *Modern Maturity, Muscle & Fitness, Natural Products News* (England), *Prime Health & Fitness,* and other publications. His original scientific articles and contributions have appeared in *Cosmetic Dermatology, Journal of the National Cancer Institute, Journal of Orthomolecular Medicine, Medical Hypotheses,* and the *New England Journal of Medicine.*

**Victoria Dolby** graduated summa cum laude from Western Oregon State College with a degree in Health Education. She writes about health issues, with a special focus on nutritional supplements, and is a regular contributor to several magazines, including *Vitamin Retailer, Better Nutrition, Natural Living Today,* and *Let's Live.* In addition, she is the managing editor of the *Nutrition Alert* newsletter and *HealthNotes Online.* Her books include *The Green Tea Book* (Avery, 1997), *Natural Therapies for Arthritis* (Keats, 1997) and *The Health Benefits of Soy* (Keats, 1996).

# HOMOCYSTEINE:
# THE SECRET KILLER

Jack Challem and Victoria Dolby

Keats Publishing, Inc.   New Canaan, Connecticut

*Homocysteine: The Secret Killer* is intended solely for
informational and educational purposes, and not as
medical advice. Please consult a medical or health
professional if you have questions about your health.

HOMOCYSTEINE: THE SECRET KILLER

**Library of Congress Cataloging-in-Publication Data**

Challem, Jack.
    Homocysteine : the secret killer / by Jack Challem and
  Victoria Dolby.
        p.      cm.
    Includes bibliographical references and index.
    ISBN 0-87983-916-3
        1. Arteriosclerosis–Etiology.    2. Homocysteine–
  Pathophysiology.    3. Vitamin B complex–Physiological effect.
  4. Cardiovascular system–Diseases–Prevention    I. Dolby, Victoria.
  II. Title.
  RC692.C448    1997
  616.1'071–dc21                                          97-39618
                                                              CIP


Printed in the United States of America

Good Health Guides are published by
Keats Publishing, Inc.
27 Pine Street (Box 876)
New Canaan, Connecticut 06840-0876

I dedicate this book to two former teachers who greatly influenced the direction of my life: DeWitt Garrett Jr., the biology professor who first introduced me to the importance of vitamins; and Harold G. Miller, my English teacher, friend, and inspiration as a writer. I cannot thank you enough. — JC

I dedicate this book to my father, William Frederick Dolby Jr. He remains a guiding force in my life. Unfortunately he died from a heart attack in 1983, before the information in this book could help him.—VD

# Contents

## A Note to Our Readers

This book is not meant to replace the professional advice of your physician. Please work with your doctor when incorporating the dietary and supplement recommendations in this book. At the very least, advise your doctor that you are adopting these recommendations.

## A Note to Physicians

As we go to press, new laboratory tests for blood and urine are becoming available to measure your patients' homocysteine levels. Based on the research, keeping their homocysteine levels in a normal range—under 6-9 micromoles per liter of blood—will reduce their risk of heart disease and stroke. For medical references documenting the role of homocysteine in disease and the protective role of folic acid and other B vitamins, please turn to the references at the back of this book.

# INTRODUCTION

## THE SECRET KILLER AND THE 2¢ CURE

AFTER YEARS OF TELLING US that high cholesterol is the cause of heart disease, and warning us to lower cholesterol levels, medicine is coming to grips with a huge and costly mistake. It turns out that cholesterol isn't the bogeyman of heart disease. The real cause of heart disease and strokes is a substance you probably never heard of until recent headlines in *Newsweek*, *TIME*, the *New York Times*, and other publications.

The secret is out, and one of the leading causes of heart disease and strokes is called homocysteine, pronounced ho´-mo-sis´-teen. If you want to dramatically lower your risk of a heart attack or stroke—and increase your chances of living to a ripe old age—you need to lower your body's levels of this dangerous substance.

How do you do that? Well, you won't find homocysteine in avoidable foods, such as eggs, meat, or fat. And you won't find dietitians recommending low-homocysteine diets. The reason is simple. Homocysteine is not found in foods.

Like cholesterol, the body makes homocysteine. It serves a brief but necessary function in the body, after which it is normally and quickly broken down or recycled back to protein. When it is not broken down, homocysteine moves through your bloodstream and slowly but surely destroys your blood vessels, laying the foundation for coronary heart disease, stroke and other cardiovascular diseases.

Amazingly, you can lower homocysteine levels—and reduce your risk of heart disease, heart attacks, and strokes—with some of the B-complex vitamins. That's right—vitamins that are cheap and easy to take.

This book tells you which vitamins and how much of them you should take. It also explains why it has taken years for this information to become known beyond a small group of physicians and researchers.

The most important of the protective vitamins is folic acid. You don't need much of it. Believe it or not, all you need is 1/70,000th of an ounce of folic acid each day. On labels of vitamins, that amount will appear as 400 mcg. It will cost you two cents a day.

Other B vitamins also play important roles in reducing homocysteine levels. Among them are vitamin B6, vitamin B12 and choline. If you take all of them in the form of a B-complex supplement—costing about ten cents a day—you'll dramatically lower your risk of heart disease, heart attacks, and strokes. You'll discover other benefits as well. You will be at a lower risk of developing cancer, you will be less depressed and have a more positive outlook in life, your mind will be sharper, and you'll feel more energized.

If all this sounds too incredible to be true, be reassured. It is true. And it is backed up by recent articles in the leading medical journals, such as the *Journal of the American Medical Association* and the *New England Journal of Medicine*. In fact, over the past several years, scientists and physicians have published more than 2,000 articles on homocysteine and the B vitamins in hundreds of medical journals. In many respects, the research on the dangers of homocysteine and the benefits of the B vitamins are better documented that the top-selling cholesterol-lowering drugs.

Certainly a very high blood level of cholesterol is a risk factor for heart disease and stroke, as are smoking, psychological stress and a lack of exercise. But many researchers and physicians have been bothered by inconsistencies in the cholesterol theory of heart disease. For example, while cholesterol is found in the fatty deposits that clog arteries, 80 percent of heart attacks occur in men with normal cholesterol levels.

Cholesterol is also essential for health, and your body makes most of what is found in your blood. It functions as an antioxidant that protects against dangerous molecules called free radicals, and it serves as a building block for your steroid hormones, which include estrogen and testosterone. You body even makes its own vitamin D from cholesterol, and this fatty substance is needed to transport vitamin E, beta-carotene and other nutrients through the blood. Without cholesterol, you would die. Indeed, several studies have found that lowering cholesterol increases the risk of cancer, suicide and, inexplicably, being murdered.

Doctors have tried to reconcile these bizarre contradictions. How can cholesterol be so important for health and yet so bad? Researchers and physicians have pointed out that there are "good" and "bad" forms of cholesterol, healthy and unhealthy ratios between the different forms of cholesterol, and, most recently, "oxidized" and "nonoxidized" cholesterol. It is almost as if they have been searching for a graceful way of admitting they've been fingering the wrong culprit all these years. For many physicians, cholesterol has gotten so confusing that they now ignore it as a cause of cardiovascular disease.

---

You might ask, if homocysteine is so dangerous and the B vitamins are so good, why haven't you heard about any of this before? That's the secret and often disturbing story of medical intrigue that we describe in this book and that Kilmer S. McCully, M.D. gives in detail in his own wonderful book, *The Homocysteine Revolution* (Keats Publishing, 1997).

The homocysteine story started innocently enough in the early 1960s when Irish researchers noted that some types of retarded children were dying of advanced heart disease or stroke before reaching puberty. The cause of this accelerated rate of cardiovascular disease turned out to be high blood levels of homocysteine.

These early medical reports intrigued McCully, then a professor of pathology at the Harvard University Medical School. He began studying the biochemical processes involving homocysteine and how this chemical caused cardiovascular disease.

In 1969, in a landmark article in the *American Journal of Pathology,* McCully proposed that high blood levels of homocysteine were not limited to a small number of retarded children. He theorized that large numbers of Americans suffered from cardiovascular disease because of elevated homocysteine levels, not cholesterol. The cure, he explained was simple: take some or all of the B-complex vitamins. Although McCully suggested all this almost 30 years ago, it is only now becoming widely accepted in medicine.

In the 1970s, however, McCully was going against the tide. Medicine was firmly committed to cholesterol as a principal cause of cardiovascular disease. Ten years later, in a medical climate antagonistic to the use of vitamins, he was fired from Harvard. Since then, McCully has continued his research on homocysteine and the B vitamins at the Veterans Administration Hospital in Providence, R.I.

Time, however, has been on McCully's side. In the early 1990s, other researchers began looking at his homocysteine theory and the roles of folic acid and other B vitamins in health. Today, McCully's research is heralded for its originality and insight.

The attention now being paid to McCully's homocysteine theory coincides with other recent and remarkable shifts in medical thinking. Over the past few years, medicine has gained a new appreciation for folic acid. It plays a fundamental role in making and repairing your deoxyribonucleic acid (DNA), the protein that composes your genes and chromosomes. Your DNA controls everything from the color of your eyes to your risk for cancer. If your DNA becomes seriously damaged, such as when you don't consume enough folic acid, your risk of developing heart disease, cancer, Alzheimer's and many other diseases increases dramatically.

The turning point occurred late in 1995, when researchers described their analysis of 38 studies on homocysteine and folic acid. In an article in the *Journal of the American Medical Association,* they reported that homocysteine was without doubt a major risk factor for cardiovascular disease. The researchers also urged Americans to increase their intake of folic acid to prevent thousands of needless deaths from heart attacks and strokes.[1]

Today, homocysteine is considered an independent risk factor for heart disease and stroke. That means it is not influenced by other risk factors, such as smoking, cholesterol and physical activity. Perhaps the most remarkable aspect of homocysteine is that it is increasingly being used as a way to identify a deficiency of folic acid. The sad fact is that such deficiencies are widespread, partly because relatively few people eat vitamin-rich fresh foods and more people eat highly processed (convenience or "fast") foods.

Just how bad is the situation? Researchers have reported that

• 59 percent of middle-age men are deficient in folic acid, 56 percent in vitamin B6, and 25 percent in vitamin B6[2];

• 30 percent of elderly men and women have elevated homocysteine levels[3]; and

• 30 to 40 percent of people with cerebrovascular and peripheral artery disease have high levels of homocysteine;[4]

The implication is astounding: the epidemic of heart diseases and stroke, which kills 40 percent of Americans, is caused in large part by not getting enough vitamins.

Furthermore, the risks of elevated homocysteine and low B vitamins are not limited to cardiovascular diseases. Physicians have long known that deficiencies of folic acid and vitamin B12 in pregnant women result in neural tube defects, such as spina bifida, in their children. Low levels of folic acid are also involved in colon cancer, prostate cancer, cervical dysplasia, diabetes and many other conditions. And vitamin B6 deficiency is often a cause of carpal tunnel syndrome.

Perhaps the most chilling recent discovery relative to homocysteine was made by separate teams of Canadian and Irish researchers. In 1995, researchers at McGill University in Montreal reported that 38 percent of Canadians had an inborn genetic defect that interfered with their utilization of folic acid.[5] Just recently, in the respected journal *Lancet*, John M. Scott, Sc.D., of Trinity College, Dublin, explained that one in every seven women has an inborn genetic defect that interferes with folic acid.[6]

The big question: do you also have this common genetic defect but don't know it? There is no easy and inexpensive way to find out—you would have to undergo genetic testing. Taking two cents' worth of folic acid supplements can compensate for this genetic defect. Supplements are also a lot easier and cheaper than genetic testing—and they can guarantee that you get enough folic acid.

---

The Food and Drug Administration, always at least one step behind the latest scientific discoveries, ordered that flours be fortified with folic acid beginning in 1998. This means more people will get folic acid when they eat bread and pastas. Although the FDA proposed food fortification of folic acid to decrease the risk of spina bifida, which affects about 2,500 newborns each year, some scientists believe that the real payoff will be a much greater decrease in cardiovascular deaths among middle-aged and elderly individuals.

But there are problems with the food fortification concept. While it is a good idea, folic acid is a fragile vitamin easily destroyed by heating. Flours are baked to make bread, and pastas are boiled, so cooking will destroy much of the folic acid added to foods.

According to Meir J. Stampfer, M.D., and Eric B. Rimm, Sc.D., of Harvard University, 86 percent of Americans consume less than 400 mcg of folic acid daily, the amount widely considered to be the minimum required to decrease the risk of cardiovascular diseases. Even with food fortification, Stampfer and Rimm pointed out, 76 percent of Americans will fall short of this amount of folic acid.[7]

Why, you might ask, haven't the big drug companies promoted the use of folic acid and the other B vitamins to prevent cardiovascular diseases? There are a couple of reasons. One is that these vitamins are no longer protected by patents and are in the public domain. That means no single company can exclusively sell and profit from them. Another reason is that vitamins, costing pennies a day, offer a meager profit compared to proprietary and patented drugs that cost people dollars a day to take. Sadly, these billion-dollar corporations are in business to make a big profit, and an inexpensive treatment for cardiovascular diseases is not in their financial interests.

In a recent issue of the *Journal of the American Medical Association*, Stampfer and Rimm, who are two of the most prominent researchers in the country, urged the U.S. government to immediately begin large-scale studies of folic acid, homocysteine, and the prevention of cardiovascular diseases. They bluntly wrote: "Because there is little commercial incentive to test such an inexpensive and nonpatentable intervention as folate [in contrast to cholesterol-lowing medication], the National Institutes of Health must step in to serve the public's interest to fund such trials. Further delays cannot be justified."[8]

----

Despite these obstacles, why is there now so much interest in homocysteine and the B vitamins? Quite simply, they have become unstoppable forces in medical research. Molecular and cell biologists now understand the detailed steps of how homocysteine causes heart attacks and strokes, and they are also showing how fundamentally important these vitamins are to our health.

Another reason is that while homocysteine tests are still expensive ($50-$100), the B-vitamin cure remains cheap. This appeals to insurance companies, which ultimately pay the medical bills of most people. They want to save money. Given the choice between spending pennies daily to prevent cardiovascular diseases versus several dollars daily to treat these diseases, it only makes sense to go the cheaper route. For this reason, you will soon see homocysteine tests becoming more routine.

In this case, cheaper is also better. It's far smarter and easier to prevent disease than to later attempt to treat it. The B vitamins are essential for health and normal components of our bodies. The discovery of homocysteine's role in causing heart attacks and strokes builds on B-vitamin research going back more than 80 years. As a natural way of preventing and treating cardiovascular diseases, folic acid and the other B vitamins are also extraordinarly safe and without side effects.

---

The rest of this book describes more about the latest research on how homocysteine causes heart disease, strokes, and other diseases. It also tells you how to preserve and improve your health with the B vitamins. After describing the research, you'll read some specific guidelines for simple changes you can make in your diet and which specific nutritional supplements to take. At the end of the book, we include specific medical journal references if you or your physician want to read the original medical studies on homocysteine, the B vitamins, and disease.

# WHAT'S WRONG WITH THE CHOLESTEROL THEORY?

CARDIOVASCULAR DISEASES KILL almost one million Americans each year—more than any other disease—and one in five Americans living today will eventually succumb to them. It's no surprise that people want to prevent and treat this deadly disease.

Cardiovascular diseases comprise a large number of conditions affecting the heart and blood vessels, including atherosclerosis, heart attack, and stroke. The condition that commonly comes to mind when discussing cardiovascular disease is coronary artery disease, which interrupts blood flow to the heart and causes a heart attack. However, many other diseases affect the heart and blood vessels.

## Some Common Types of Cardiovascular Diseases

### Angina
Chest pain is the primary symptom of angina, a condition in which the heart muscle does not receive adequate blood supply.
### Arteriosclerosis
This is a general term for the process commonly known as hardening of the arteries.

### Atherosclerosis
A form of arteriosclerosis in which fatty deposits of plaque block blood flow in medium and large arteries.

### Coronary artery disease
Hardening of the arteries that supply blood to the heart muscle, often the cause of a heart attack.

**Embolism**
Obstruction of blood flow by a blood clot, air bubble, or foreign material.

**Heart attack**
Myocardial infarction, the technical term for a heart attack, occurs when the blood flow to the heart is severely limited or stopped.

**Hypertension**
Blood pressure readings above 140/90 are considered high and indicate that the heart and arteries are under excessive strain. Also known as high blood pressure.

**Peripheral artery disease**
Narrowing of the blood vessels in the legs and arms, usually as a result of atherosclerosis.

**Stroke**
Brain damage caused by a ruptured or blocked blood vessel in the brain.

**Thrombosis**
A blood clot.

Early research identified cardiovascular disease risk factors by searching for common traits and lifestyles in people afflicted with disease. These risk factors include being male, increasing age, family history of disease, elevated cholesterol levels, hypertension, tobacco use, diabetes, obesity, stress, oral contraceptive use, excessive alcohol intake, malnutrition, and lack of physical activity.

Cholesterol quickly took center stage as the most important risk factor in the development of cardiovascular diseases. But cholesterol may not be the real culprit.

## CHOLESTEROL'S BAD REPUTATION

Walk down the aisle of any grocery store and you'll notice the words "low cholesterol," "no cholesterol," and "cholesterol free," plastered on bottles, boxes, and bags. Cholesterol has become the villain of cardiovascular disease—avoid it and you can dodge this dreaded killer. So they say.

Despite all the fuss, cholesterol per se may not be all that important as a cause of cardiovascular disease. Cholesterol, produced by our bodies and present in every single cell, performs many functions essential for health. For example, one type of cholesterol acts as a building block for steroid hormones, such as sexual hormones, and another is converted into vitamin D when the skin is exposed to sunlight. Cholesterol is also important during the metabolism of carbohydrates, for the transportation of fat-soluble vitamins (such as vitamins A and E and beta-carotene) in the bloodstream, as a raw material for building cell membranes, and even as an antioxidant protecting against free radical damage.

Cholesterol did not have a bad rap until 1913. That's when a Russian scientist named Nikolai Anitschkow fed a group of rabbits a very high cholesterol diet as an experiment. When Anitschkow examined the rabbits' blood vessels, he found them to be clogged with plaque, a condition known as atheroslerosis. Since the addition of cholesterol was the only significant change in the lives of these animals, he concluded that cholesterol was the cause of their cardiovascular disease.

Researchers subsequently hypothesized that more cholesterol in the diet translated into more cholesterol in the blood. This extra cholesterol settled onto the blood-vessel walls and formed fatty buildups called plaques, which eventually blocked the normal flow of blood. If a clot formed where a plaque had accumulated, blood flow would be completely blocked, causing a heart attack or stroke.

However, this turn-of-the-century study contained serious weaknesses when examined under the strict scrutiny of modern research. For example, the rabbits—which are essentially vegetarian animals—were fed a cholesterol-rich diet equivalent to a person eating 50 eggs daily. It was probably unreasonable to expect vegetarian rabbits to metabolize such large amounts of animal fat.

Another problem with applying Anitschkow's study to human cardiovascular disease is that the type of arteriosclerosis developed by these rabbits was different from that afflicting modern man. This weakens the assumption that a cholesterol-rich diet in rabbits that causes a cardiovascular disease is the culprit in our health epidemic.

## UPDATING THE CHOLESTEROL THEORY

Problems abound with the cholesterol model of cardiovascular disease. Cholesterol is essential to life, and most of the cholesterol in the bloodstream is manufactured by the liver rather than being the result of eating meat, eggs, and dairy products. In fact, only about one-third of blood cholesterol can be traced to dietary sources.

Not surprisingly, a number of researchers have pointed out that avoiding cholesterol-rich foods has only a limited effect on lowering total cholesterol levels. So the cholesterol we eat does not necessarily result in the cholesterol that builds up on our blood vessel walls. Today, many Americans feel so overwhelmed by the sheer amount of information about cholesterol and cardiovascular disease that they have given up on understanding the issue.

## LIPOPROTEIN SHUTTLES

In an effort to reconcile the inconsistencies of the cholesterol theory of cardiovascular disease, many scientists have focused their attention on the role of different types of cholesterol. Since cholesterol is fat-based, it must be wrapped in water-soluble bubbles, called lipoproteins, to shuttle it through the bloodstream. There are several kinds of lipoprotein ferries. The ones most people are familiar with are low density lipoprotein (LDL) and high density lipoprotein (HDL).

Lipoproteins perform slightly different functions in the body. For example, LDL transports more cholesterol than the HDL. However, the LDLs tend to keep the cholesterol in the blood, while HDL shuttles it back to the liver to be broken down and excreted from the body. Therefore, higher levels of HDL will actually help lower total cholesterol levels.

## THE NUMBERS GAME

Scientists have theorized that the ratio between different types of cholesterol is more important to cardiovascular disease risk than total cholesterol levels alone. Thus, the concept of LDL as the "bad cholesterol" and HDL as the "good cholesterol" was born. Public health officials have urged people to lower their LDL levels and raise their HDL levels to prevent cardiovascular diseases.

According to the National Cholesterol Education Program, the risk of cardiovascular disease is moderate when:
• Total blood cholesterol is more than 200 mg per deciliter of blood, and
• LDL cholesterol is more than 130 mg per deciliter.

And, accordingly, a high risk of cardiovascular disease occurs when:
• Total blood cholesterol is more than 220 mg. per deciliter, and
• LDL cholesterol is more than 160 mg per deciliter.

The National Cholesterol Education Program also states that the lowest risk of cardiovascular disease is found in individuals with a ratio of total cholesterol to HDL cholesterol below 3.5 to 1, moderate risk begins at a ratio of 4.5 to 1, and high risk starts at a ratio of 6.5 to 1. For example, if your total cholesterol level is 225 and your HDL cholesterol is 50, you have a ratio of 4.5 to 1, indicating a moderate risk of developing cardiovascular disease.

Unfortunately, several studies show that just keeping tabs on your total cholesterol level or your LDL/HDL ratios is not necessarily a surefire way to avoid cardiovascular disease. Heart attacks, unfortunately, often strike men and women with "normal" cholesterol levels and ratios.

## OTHER CARDIOVASCULAR RISK FACTORS

Needless to say, doctors were stumped by the cholesterol inconsistencies. Some of their patients had enviably low cholesterol levels, yet they still suffered heart attacks or other cardiovascular diseases. Pieces of the cardiovascular disease puzzle were obviously missing.

In the continuing search for answers, some researchers have focused on the effects of free radical damage to cholesterol. Free radicals are highly reactive molecules found in tobacco smoke and air pollution and are produced in the body during normal metabolic processes. Free radicals are unstable because they have an unpaired electron. As a result, they readily rob healthy molecules of an electron to replace the missing one. The consequence is called oxidation, and which can cause severe damage to the body, much in the same way oxygen turns butter rancid.

Several recent studies indicate that one of the prime targets of free radicals is LDL cholesterol. And once LDL is oxidized it becomes a very nasty substance. Scientists had already; implicated nonoxidized LDL in the initiation of arteriosclerosis, now they realized that oxidized LDL was even more likely to damage blood vessels and promote cardiovascular disease. Interestingly, homocysteine may also cause oxidative damage to LDL.[9, 10] The antioxidant vitamins (vitamins C, E, and beta-carotene) show a great deal of promise in preventing the oxidation of LDL, and thus reducing this cardiovascular disease risk factor.

Another type of lipoprotein, known as lipoprotein(a), or Lp(a), is very similar to LDL. Elevated levels of Lp(a) in the blood increase the risk of several cardiovascular diseases, including coronary artery disease, stroke and atherosclerosis, according to Ernst J. Schaefer, M.D. and colleagues at the Lipid Metabolism Laboratory, U.S. Department of Agriculture Human Nutrition Center on Aging at Tufts University, Boston. Some researchers now recognize high levels of Lp(a) as an independent risk factor for cardiovascular diseases, especially in individuals who also have high cholesterol levels. Lp(a) can also be made more dangerous to the heart and blood vessels if it is oxidized by free radicals.[11]

## Risk Factors for Cardiovascular Diseases

**You can change...**
>   Diet
>   Tobacco use
>   Cholesterol levels
>   Blood pressure
>   Exercise level
>   Obesity
>   Stress level

**You cannot change...**
>   Age
>   Gender
>   Heredity
>   Diabetes

Most risk factors for cardiovascular diseases are well within your control.

# THE HOMOCYSTEINE THEORY OF CARDIOVASCULAR DISEASE

THE CONVENTIONAL cardiovascular disease risk factors, such as high cholesterol levels, smoking, and hypertension cannot completely account for why cardiovascular diseases are the number one killer of Americans. In fact, Johan B. Ubbink, Sc.D., a cardiovascular disease researcher at the Department of Chemical Pathology, University of Pretoria, South Africa, recently noted that the most commonly recognized risk factors—despite being studied exhaustively—explain only about 50 percent of all cases of cardiovascular disease.[8] Clearly there are other, unrecognized causes of cardiovascular disease. Scientists are making an effort to identify these additional causes; many consider elevated homocysteine to be a cause and call it the "new cholesterol."

You've probably heard little or nothing about homocysteine. But, if you suffer from a cardiovascular disease, there's a good chance that your homocysteine levels are elevated. Unfortunately, your doctor has probably never checked your homocysteine levels. Furthermore, your doctor may not even know what homocysteine is or how easy it is to lower its level with the B vitamins.

Fortunately, a growing number of doctors are beginning to recognize–and test patients for–a high homocysteine level as an independent risk factor for cardiovascular diseases.

## WHAT IS HOMOCYSTEINE?

If elevated homocysteine is so strongly associated with

cardiovascular disease, you may be wondering why no one has demanded that it be banned from the marketplace or established a health education program to get people to eat less of it. The answer is simple: homocysteine is not sold in stores and is not found in foods. Homocysteine, like cholesterol, is produced naturally in the human body. Unlike cholesterol, homocysteine is supposed to exist only briefly before the body converts it into either useful or harmless substances.

Protein, particularly the essential amino acid methionine (found in meat), is the indirect source of homocysteine. When the body digests and metabolizes methionine, it produces homocysteine before either recycling methionine or creating the final breakdown product, cystathionine.

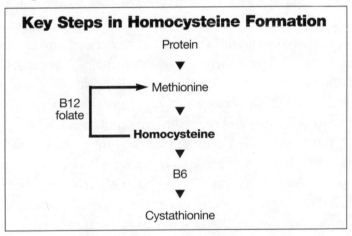

## Key Steps in Homocysteine Formation

Protein
▼

B12 folate

Methionine
▼
Homocysteine
▼
B6
▼
Cystathionine

There are many circumstances in which homocysteine becomes a long-lived, potentially deadly byproduct of protein metabolism. For example, an inadequate supply of key B vitamins "freezes" homocysteine metabolism before it is converted to cystathionine. When this happens, abnormally high levels of homocysteine build up in the bloodstream and damage blood vessels. This condition is known as homocysteinemia.

Abnormal levels of homocysteine can damage any and all of the body's blood vessels. When the blood vessels feeding the heart are damaged; this is called coronary artery disease. When the blood vessels that nourish the brain are affected, stroke is the likely outcome. And if the blood vessels of the hands or legs are affected, peripheral artery disease is the likely consequence.

## SOLVING THE CARDIOVASCULAR DISEASE MYSTERY

The story of homocysteine's discovery as a risk factor for cardiovascular disease reads like a mystery novel. The first chapter began in 1962 at the Royal Belfast Hospital for Sick Children in Northern Ireland. The first sleuths on the scene were Dr. Nina Carson and her colleagues, who were investigating how biochemical disorders influence severe forms of mental retardation. Carson knew that genetically linked enzyme deficiencies could be a red flag for retardation, so she was screening at-risk families for a wide range of enzyme deficiencies.

During this biochemical screening she analyzed the urine of two severely retarded sisters, ages four and six. Both of these girls lacked normal function of an enzyme needed during amino acid metabolism. This unusual condition is characterized by the excretion of homocystine (an oxidized form of homocysteine) in the urine. This struck the doctors as strange because homocystine is not usually present in the urine. Soon after these two cases were recorded, the doctors found several other young retarded patients with the same enzyme deficiency, which Dr. Carson called homocystinuria.

About three years after the discovery of homocystinuria, the older sister died. An autopsy unexpectedly revealed severe atherosclerosis. It was as if this nine-year-old girl had the hardened blood vessels of an old woman. The autopsies on other young casualties of homocystinuria in subsequent years found the same accelerated process of cardiovascular disease.

Since this type of homocystinuria only affects about one in 200,000 individuals, it was initially considered a rare disease. The discovery of premature cardiovascular disease in retarded children would have remained a medical oddity had it not been for another doctor who made a startling connection between homocysteine levels and cardiovascular diseases among the general public.

## THE NEXT PUZZLE PIECE

Kilmer McCully, M.D., currently a pathologist at the Veterans Administration Hospital in Providence, R.I., was a researcher in genetics and molecular biology at Harvard Medical School in 1969. It was in that year that McCully became aware of a case report of a boy afflicted with homocystinuria. This boy died when he was eight years old, and an autopsy found arteries clogged with plaque; the cause of death was stroke. McCully became fascinated with the pathology of homocystinuria when he learned of yet another fatal case of this disease, this time in a two-month-old baby who died from severe atherosclerosis.

McCully published a provocative scientific paper in the *American Journal of Pathology* in which he described the possible link between children with homocystinuria, individuals with other enzyme deficiencies, and cardiovascular disease. The cases he wrote about in this article all had two striking, significant commonalties: unusually high levels of homocysteine and arterial damage leading to atherosclerosis.[13]

McCully concluded that there was a cause-and-effect

relationship—that abnormal levels of homocysteine caused cardiovascular disease. He proposed that even normal individuals, without enzyme deficiencies, could develop dangerous levels of homocysteine, and subsequently cardiovascular diseases, under certain circumstances, such as vitamin deficiencies.

## THE VITAMIN LINK

Fitting together the puzzle pieces in this emerging homocysteine mystery required two steps. First, researchers identified a pattern between unusual levels of homocysteine and premature cardiovascular disease in children with enzyme disorders. Second, researchers realized that certain dietary deficiencies caused a dangerous increase in homocysteine levels in normal adults. As it turned out, this dietary link had been discovered 20 years earlier.

In 1949, researchers investigated the role of B vitamins in a group of monkeys fed diets deficient in different nutrients. When the monkeys' diets lacked vitamin B6, but were adequate in all other nutrients, they developed atherosclerosis. Although this study was widely reported, most scientists were unable to fit this information in with the prevailing cholesterol theory of cardiovascular disease. As a result, the findings were dismissed as interesting, but unimportant. The significance of this study would not be realized until McCully began investigating homocysteine.

McCully knew that vitamin B6 is essential for complete metabolism of the amino acid methionine. Homocysteine is created during the breakdown of methionine, but vitamin B6 converts homocysteine into harmless cystathionine. McCully hypothesized that the vitamin B6 deficient monkeys developed high homocysteine levels, which then resulted in atherosclerosis. This connection has become the cornerstone of the homocysteine theory of cardiovascular disease: that unnatural accumulation of homocysteine in the blood causes atherosclerosis, whereas adequate intake of B vitamins allows normal metabolism of homocysteine and reduces the risk of cardiovascular disease.

# HOW HOMOCYSTEINE CAUSES CARDIOVASCULAR DISEASE

AFTER MAKING THE CONNECTION between abnormal homocysteine levels and cardiovascular disease, McCully decided that it was time to put his theory to the test. In one of his first experiments, he cultured some skin cells taken from an individual who lacked an enzyme that helped remove homocysteine from the body. Ordinarily, skin cells produce a fibrous substance called proteoglycan. However, the proteoglycan from enzyme-lacking skin cells produced a grainy (diseased) rather than fibrous (healthy) substance.

Also, when homocysteine was added to normal skin cells, the same grainy substance replaced the ordinarily fibrous proteoglycan. McCully proposed that high levels of homocysteine in the blood initiate arteriosclerosis by changing the fibrous substance produced by proteoglycans in blood vessel walls, much the way this happens in the skin.

McCully's next experiment went beyond cells grown in laboratory dishes. He injected rabbits with either homocysteine or a placebo every 12 hours for up to 35 days. The rabbits were also fed diets containing different amounts of vitamin B6 and cholesterol. By the end of the experiment, the rabbits injected with homocysteine developed arteriosclerotic plaque, whereas the rabbits injected with the placebo had normal blood vessel walls. McCully noted that the location and characteristics of the plaques formed in the homocysteine-injected rabbits were very similar to the plaques seen in humans with arteriosclerosis.

Cardiovascular disease developed very quickly in the rabbits exposed to homocysteine—in as short a time as 20 days. Even more significantly, the amount of homocysteine leading to arteriosclerotic plaque in the rabbits was comparable to the amount of homocysteine produced by people eating typical dietary amounts of methionine in protein-containing foods.

Only moderately elevated levels of homocysteine were required to produce arteriosclerosis in rabbits. This finding suggested that the amount of homocysteine produced from an average human diet could, in the right circumstances, lead to cardiovascular disease. In contrast, the 1913 rabbit study that identified cholesterol as the cause of cardiovascular disease was based on an unrealistic cholesterol level equivalent to what would be obtained by the consumption of 50 eggs a day in a human diet.

McCully's study, however, did find that cholesterol played a role in cardiovascular disease—but only after homocysteine began damaging blood vessels. Specifically, he found that adding cholesterol to the diets of some of the homocysteine-exposed rabbits resulted in the buildup of fatty material on blood vessel walls. Significantly, these fatty deposits were also associated with the homocysteine-altered proteoglycans. The homocysteine damage to blood vessel walls preceded the cholesterol-based atherosclerotic plaques.

Another animal experiment was undertaken by McCully to confirm these findings. Rabbits were divided into groups fed normal diets supplemented with homocysteine or a placebo. The homocysteine levels were comparable to a human diet containing about five times the daily requirement of the amino acid methionine—not an unusual amount among Americans. The rabbits exposed to this amount of homocysteine developed thickened, plaque-filled arteries.[14]

A microscopic examination of cells extracted from the rabbits' plaques found them to be similar to the blood vessel injuries in children with homocystinuria. The higher the dosage of the homocysteine and the longer the rabbits were exposed to homocysteine, the more severe were their blood vessel injuries. In fact, almost 60 percent of the rabbits on the highest homocysteine dosages died within four to eight weeks. Their autopsies revealed massive blood clots in the blood vessels of the lungs which fatally blocked the flow of blood. Amazingly, none of the rabbits developed blood clots or died prematurely when supplemented with vitamin B6.

In another experiment, rabbits were fed diets generally believed to cause cardiovascular disease. They were given a basic laboratory diet, but with butter and cholesterol, rather than homocysteine, added to their feed. The rabbits had fewer and less severe blood vessel injuries than the homocysteine-fed rabbits.

These homocysteine studies helped uncover the chain of events underlying the development of arteriosclerosis. First, too little vitamin B6 in relation to the amount of methionine in the diet reduces the body's ability to metabolize homocysteine. Homocysteine levels in the bloodstream build up because protein metabolism is "stuck" at this step.

Second, the homocysteine in the blood attacks and strips away areas of the blood vessel walls. These injured, bare patches—perhaps in the body's misguided attempts at healing—are filled in with cholesterol and other fatty substances, a process known as arteriosclerosis. These diseased patches, called atheromas, expand and injure passing blood cells, causing them to clot. These clots, known as thromboses, can block blood flow, causing a heart attack or stroke.

---

## Chain of Events in the Development of Cardiovascular Disease

Low intake of B vitamins or high intake of methionine

▼

Build up of homocysteine

▼

Proteoglycans in blood vessels release abnormal substances

▼

Blood-vessel walls damaged

▼

Fatty deposits of plaque accumulate
in damaged areas of blood-vessel walls

▼

Cholesterol deposits grow on damaged areas

▼

Blood clots may form

▼

Heart attack or stroke

---

## A CLOSER LOOK AT HOMOCYSTEINE IN THE BLOOD VESSELS

The mechanism by which homocysteine alters the structure of blood vessel walls is complex. The cells that line the arteries and other blood vessels produce proteoglycans (the same substance studied in the skin-cell experiments discussed earlier). Proteoglycans are made up of many carbohydrate molecules surrounding a protein core.

In the presence of homocysteine, proteoglycans in the blood vessel walls lose the ability to cross-link and create their normal fibrous structure. The homocysteine-altered proteoglycans take on a more granular form of organization, and these abnormal proteoglycans are likely to aggregate into clumps in the bloodstream. Lipoproteins flowing in the bloodstream bind to these dissolved proteoglycans, which then are deposited into the blood vessel linings as plaque.[15]

McCully studied the effects of homocysteine at Harvard Medical School for about 10 years. However, this insightful research almost came to a grinding halt in 1979. Believing McCully had failed to prove his homocysteine theory, his department head fired him. It took McCully two years to find a job as a pathologist at the Veterans Administration Hospital in Providence, R.I. His hard work was being ignored by a scientific community focusing only on the better-known risk factors in cardiovascular diseases. But being an outcast did not stop McCully. He continued to research the role of homocysteine and B vitamins in cardiovascular diseases. Today, he has been proved right: the medical community embraces McCully's research and finally acknowledges the important role that homocysteine plays in cardiovascular diseases.

## PROVING THE CASE FOR HOMOCYSTEINE

Homocysteine remained on the scientific back burner for at least a decade after McCully left Harvard. By the late 1980s and early 1990s, signs began emerging that linked homocysteine and intake of the B vitamins to cardiovascular disease— signs that even the skeptical scientific community could no longer ignore.

A 1992 study, led by Meir J. Stampfer, M.D., a professor of epidemiology and nutrition at Harvard Medical School—the very institution that dismissed McCully's theory that homocysteine plays a causative role in cardiovascular disease—analyzed data from the Physicians Health Study. This study of approximately 15,000 doctors revealed strong evidence that homocysteine does indeed influence cardiovascular disease. Stampfer found that men with homocysteine levels 12 percent above average had a whopping 3.4-fold greater risk of having a heart attack than men with low levels, regardless of other cardiovascular disease risk factors.[16]

McCully, in a 1988 study, measured the levels of homocysteine in the blood serum of people with and without coronary artery disease. Homocysteine levels in people with coronary artery disease were ten times higher than in people without cardiovascular disease![17]

A more recent study, published in the 1995 *New England Journal of Medicine*, sought to answer two questions: One, is homocysteinemia (high blood levels of homocysteine) really predictive of cardiovascular disease? And two, how many people have unhealthy homocysteine levels? The answer to the first question, according to Robert Clarke, M.R.C.P.I., of Adelaide Hospital in Ireland, is *yes*, homocysteine is linked to the development of heart disease. As for the second question, only two percent of the general, healthy population have high levels of homocysteine, but about 30 percent of patients with cardiovascular diseases have abnormally elevated homocysteine levels.[18]

Specifically, 42 percent of the patients suffering from cerebrovascular disease (affecting the blood vessels of the brain), 28 percent of patients with peripheral artery disease (affecting the blood vessels of the arms and legs), and 30 percent of patients with coronary artery disease (affecting the blood vessels of the heart) had very high blood levels of homocysteine. None of the 27 randomly chosen men and women free of cardiovascular diseases, but who were tested for the sake of comparison, had abnormal homocysteine levels. The researchers concluded that homocysteine is up to 40 times more predictive than cholesterol in assessing cardiovascular disease risk. This means it is far more important to know your homocysteine than your cholesterol levels.

## HOMOCYSTEINE AND HEART ATTACKS

A study published by Bo Israelsson, M.D., of the Malmö General Hospital, Sweden, examined homocysteine levels in a group of men who had their first heart attack at a relatively young age.[19] By most measures, these men, all under age 55, were at low risk of suffering a heart attack. Their blood pressure, cholesterol and triglyceride levels were normal, and none had ever shown any previous sign of cardiovascular disease. Nevertheless, they all experienced "premature" heart attacks. This prompted some researchers to search for a hidden cardiovascular disease risk factor linking these men.

As it turned out, about a quarter of the men had high levels of homocysteine. Israelsson wrote in the journal *Atherosclerosis* that "this study confirms that moderate homocysteinemia exists in a high proportion of men with low conventional risk factors for arteriosclerotic disease, who, despite low risk factors, develop [heart attacks] at an early age." Similarly, the men with abnormal homocysteine levels had subnormal or low blood concentrations of folic acid, a B vitamin important in the metabolism of homocysteine. Their levels of vitamin B12 were also in the lower range of normal. This correlation between high homocysteine levels and low levels of B vitamins appears to be the missing link accounting for many "unexplained" heart attacks.

A recent study, conducted by Dr. Paul N. Hopkins at the University of Utah School of Medicine, Salt Lake City, found that men with a family history of heart disease and elevated levels of homocysteine have a 14-fold higher risk of developing hardened arteries in their hearts (a common cause of heart attacks), the same situation in women increases their risk 13-fold.[20]

## HOMOCYSTEINE AND STROKES

Strokes are a type of cardiovascular disease that can result in brain damage or even death. They are caused by a lack of blood supply to the brain due to a blocked or ruptured blood vessel. Several studies have reported that high homocysteine levels increase the risk of stroke. For example, 421 patients with cardiovascular disease were recently screened for homocysteinemia. Twenty percent of the men and women diagnosed with cerebral occlusive arterial disease were found to have mildly elevated levels of homocysteine, indicating that they were at an increased risk of having a stroke.[21]

Another study, published in the journal *Stroke,* compared the homocysteine levels of 72 patients who either had suffered from a stroke or had the risk factors for a stroke to 31 normal individuals.[22] The stroke patients had significantly higher homocysteine levels compared with the normal group. The researchers concluded that elevated homocysteine was a major risk factor for stroke.

## HOMOCYSTEINE AND PERIPHERAL ARTERY DISEASE

Arteriosclerosis, or hardening of the arteries, can develop in any of the arteries of the body. When it occurs in the arteries supplying blood to the lower extremities or arms, it is known as peripheral artery disease. Intermittent claudication (pain and cramping in the legs) is a common symptom of peripheral artery disease.

Homocysteine has been suggested as a significant risk factor in peripheral artery disease. One clinical trial conducted at the Oregon Health Sciences University in Portland, Oregon by Manuel Rene Malinow, M.D. compared the homocysteine levels between 47 patients with peripheral artery disease and 103 healthy subjects.[23] After taking into account differences that could be caused by age, the researchers found that homocysteine levels were significantly higher in the group suffering from peripheral artery disease. Another study, based on 214 patients with cardiovascular disease and a group of controls, reported that peripheral artery disease progresses more quickly in individuals with high homocysteine levels than in those with normal blood levels.[24]

## GENETIC RISKS

Many enzymes, or catalysts, are involved in the complete metabolism of homocysteine. If any of these enzymes is defective or functions inefficiently, the body is less able to successfully process homocysteine. Dr. Paul W. Wong at the University of Chicago recently reported that many people have inefficient forms of several key enzymes needed in this process, which allows their homocysteine levels—and risk of cardiovascular disease—to rise.[25]

Dr. Rima Rozen, a geneticist at McGill University in Montreal, was able to identify the mutated gene that leads to the enzyme inefficiency noted by Wong. Furthermore, Rozen found that while one in two people carries one copy of the defective gene, 12 percent of people have two copies of the gene (one from each parent), which results in abnormally high homocysteine levels. Other studies have found that inborn genetic defects in folic acid affect somewhere between 14 and 38 percent of people. The risk of genetic defects further compromising folic acid utilization increases with age, because aging entails an increase in DNA damage. The genetic test to identify this defective enzyme is not yet available to the general public, but should be in the near future.

The consequence of this genetic defect is that even if you obtain "normal" levels of folic acid through the diet, they may not be enough to control homocysteine. The sluggish gene and enzyme prevent the body from converting dietary folic acid to 5-methytetrahydrofolate, the form of the nutrient found in the blood. More folic acid, suggested Wong and other researchers, improves the enzyme's efficiency and raises blood levels of the vitamin.

## CONCLUSIVE EVIDENCE

The *Journal of the American Medical Association* is the 500-pound gorilla of medical journals, and on October 4, 1995, it weighed in with one of the most compelling studies of homocysteine and heart disease. A "meta," or collective, analysis of 38 previous studies found homocysteine did play a causative role in cardiovascular disease—while the B-vitamin folic acid was protective.[26]

According to the principal researcher, Carol J. Boushey, Ph.D., currently at Southern Illinois University in Carbondale, this study examined 209 relevant scientific studies conducted during a recent six-year span of time. She and her colleagues focused their attention on 27 studies relating to homocysteine in the development of cardiovascular disease and 11 on the effect of folic acid on homocysteine levels. Of the 17 studies that dealt specifically with homocysteine in coronary artery disease, 14 showed that the risk of this cardiovascular disease rose hand in hand with homocysteine levels. Similarly, 9 of the 11 studies that included data on cerebrovascular disease showed a causal relationship between homocysteine and stroke, and 9 trials implicated homocysteine in peripheral artery disease.

Folic acid emerged from this study as a nutritional star. There was a clear inverse relationship between folic acid and homocysteine in the blood, meaning that as levels of folic acid in the blood rose, levels of homocysteine dropped. Several of the studies examined by Boushey reported that folic acid supplementation lowered homocysteine levels, even in people who were not deficient in this B vitamin. In some of the studies high doses of folic acid (i.e. as much as 10,000 mcg) were administered; however, much smaller doses of folic acid showed a remarkable ability to lower abnormal homocysteine levels. For example, 650 mcg of folic acid cut homocysteine concentrations by 42 percent.

The other B vitamins were also found to play a role in lowering homocysteine levels. Vitamins B6 and B12 both showed a significant effect on elevated homocysteine levels. "Folic acid, on the other hand," Boushey notes, "seems to be the key factor in reducing [high homocysteine levels]."

High levels of homocysteine were conservatively estimated to be responsible for as many as one in every ten deaths from coronary artery disease in American men over age 45—about 35,000 men every year. In women, homocysteine accounted for about 6 percent, or 21,000, fatal heart attacks.

Many, if not all, of these homocysteine-related cardio-vascular disease fatalities are preventable. Boushey suggested three ways in which Americans could increase their intake of folic acid in order to reduce the cardiovascular disease time bomb of elevated homocysteine levels.

• First, two or three additional servings of folic acid-rich fruits and vegetables could be added to the daily diet. Since only half of the folic acid from foods is used by the body, this would have the smallest effect on cardiovascular disease prevention.

• Second, Americans could supplement with 400 mcg of folic acid daily. This level of supplementation would lower the risk of cardiovascular disease slightly more than someone cutting total cholesterol by 20 mg/dL. If only half of those with high homocysteine levels supplemented with folic acid, the reduced risk of heart attack and stroke would be similar to 80 percent of Americans increasing their fruit and vegetable intake.

• Third, folic acid could be fortified in the food supply, much in the way that vitamin D is currently added to milk. If 350 mcg of folic acid were added to flour and cereal, Boushey estimated that "the deaths of more than 30,000 men and 19,000 women might be prevented.

"A strong case therefore can be made for the inference that increased folic acid intake could prevent arteriosclerotic vascular disease. Controlled trials with folic acid would be the most convincing proof. Such trials would require many years to show results. In the meantime, policies for increasing folic acid intake could have a considerable effect on the prevention of arteriosclerotic vascular disease," Boushey concluded.

On the heels of this powerful study came another homocysteine trial showing homocysteine to be a major risk factor for cardiovascular disease. This study, published in the *International Journal of Epidemiology,* examined the relationship of homocysteine levels to the risk of heart attacks in 21,826 men and women. Dr. Egil Arnesen, of the Institute of Community Medicine, University of Tromsø, Norway, found that "...there is no threshold level below which homocysteine is not associated with risk of myocardial infarction. A considerable proportion of the population may therefore be at risk due to elevated serum homocysteine level."[29] And the studies just keep rolling in. Howard I. Morrison, Ph.D. and colleagues at the Laboratory Centre for Disease Control in Canada measure folic acid levels in 5,056 middle-aged men and women and recorded how many of these people later died of heart disease. As it turned out, those with the lowest folic acid levels were much more likely to have a fatal heart attack. But even those with levels of folic acid in the "normal" range had an increased risk for cardiovascular disease. Consequently, Morrison urged that the definition of what is "normal" for folic acid needs to be reassessed, since higher levels are obviously required to lessen the risk of heart disease.[28]

There seems to be no bounds to the positive things scientists have to say about the potential of folic acid to save lives. Robert M. Russell, M.D., of Tufts University, after reviewing the body of literature, wrote in the *Journal of the American Medical Association* that increasing folic acid intake to 400 mcg daily would conservatively save 13,500 lives each year—individuals who would otherwise die from homocysteine-related heart disease.[29] Isn't it amazing that such a simple dietary addition has such potential to save lives?

# Milestones in the Homocysteine Theory of Cardiovascular Disease

## Identifying the Problem:
- Young retarded children found to have abnormal levels of homocysteine in their urine, which results in the surprisingly early and fatal development of arteriosclerosis.

- Animal studies confirm that homocysteine, in animals and human cells, can cause cardiovascular diseases.

- High homocysteine levels found to be more common in those suffering from strokes, heart attacks, and other cardiovascular diseases than healthy individuals.

- High levels of homocysteine are discovered to be prevalent in individuals lacking sufficient amounts of B vitamins.

## Finding the Solution:
- Supplements of certain B vitamins (folic acid, vitamin B6, vitamin B12, choline, and/or betaine) are found to reduce dangerously high levels of homocysteine.

- Lowering homocysteine levels reduces the risk of heart attack, stroke, and other cardiovascular diseases.

# THE BENEFICIAL
# ROLE OF B VITAMINS

ALMOST HALF A CENTURY AGO, researchers initiated the longest-running cardiovascular disease study, involving 5,209 residents of Framingham, Massachusetts. This "Framingham Heart Study" continues today, with the surviving original members and a second generation of subjects. Recently, researchers from Tufts University in Boston examined homocysteine levels, vitamin status, and cardiovascular disease in 1,000 of the original Framingham men.[30]

The Tufts University researchers used ultrasound to measure how well blood was flowing through the carotid arteries (the major blood vessels feeding blood to the head and brain) of these men. When fatty deposits of plaque build up on the linings of these important blood vessels (a condition known as carotid artery stenosis), the opening of the arteries can be significantly narrowed and obstruct blood flow. If these arteries are narrowed by 25 percent or more, the risk of stroke or coronary artery disease is greatly increased.

Previous research in the Framingham Heart Study had already demonstrated a link between elevated homocysteine levels and low levels of the B vitamins folic acid, vitamin B6, and vitamin B12 in these men. This investigation focused on whether there was also a link between homocysteine and cardiovascular disease.

When the extent of carotid artery narrowing was compared with homocysteine and vitamin status, the researchers found that the men with the most severe arterial blockage had the highest homocysteine levels and lowest B vitamin levels. These men were, consequently, at the greatest risk of having a stroke or heart attack.

The researchers were surprised to find that "normal" levels of homocysteine caused cardiovascular disease, which "require[s] us to reconsider the current definition of elevated homocysteine concentrations." If normal levels lead to a heart attack or stroke, it's definitely time to reconsider the meaning of normal and acceptable homocysteine levels.

Since "two thirds of all cases of elevated homocysteine concentrations were associated with inadequate concentrations of one of more of these vitamins," i.e., folic acid, vitamin B6, and vitamin B12, the way to avoid heart attacks or strokes seems clear. Simply reduce homocysteine levels by maintaining adequate B vitamin intake.

The lead researcher of this study, Jacob Selhub, Ph.D., explained to *The Saturday Evening Post* (May/June 1995) that very tiny amounts of homocysteine in the blood can have an incredible impact on cardiovascular health. To give some perspective, Selhub said that homocysteine is present in the blood at one-thousandth of the concentration of cholesterol. As little as a 20 to 30 percent increase in this minuscule amount of homocysteine can greatly increase the risk of cardiovascular disease.

## A CLASSIC INVERSE RELATIONSHIP

In an inverse relationship, the increase of one event causes another event to decrease—kind of like the motion of a seesaw. For example, with homocysteine and the B vitamins, increasing intake of B vitamins lowers homocysteine levels. The reverse is also true: homocysteine levels increase when B vitamin intake is low. Selhub demonstrated this inverse relationship between folic acid, vitamin B12, and vitamin B6 and homocysteine in a recent study based on the data from 1,160 participants in the Framingham Heart Study. Selhub reported that an astonishing "67% of the cases of high homocysteine" could be traced to low levels of one or more of the B vitamins.[31]

A majority of men and women with low blood levels of folate (another name for folic acid) will see their homocysteine levels creep up. Up to 84 percent of individuals with folate deficiencies and 56 percent with borderline folate serum concentrations have high homocysteine levels, according to Soo-Sang Kang, M.D., Ph.D., of Rush-Presbyterian-St. Luke's Medical Center in Chicago. "All subjects with subnormal serum folate showed more than 1.65-fold increase of serum total homocyst(e)ine," states Kang, "suggesting that a depletion of folic acid was primarily responsible for the accumulation of homocyst(e)ine."[32]

Researchers at the Centers for Disease Control and Prevention in Atlanta recently took advantage of the clear relationship between folic acid and homocysteine to indirectly investigate homocysteine as a stroke risk factor. As lead researcher Wayne H. Giles, M.D., M.S., explains, "homocyst(e)ine levels were not obtained on the participants in the First National Health and Nutrition Examination Survey (NHANES I). However, serum folate levels were obtained on a subset of NHANES I participants." Therefore, folic acid levels, as an indirect assessment of homocysteine concentrations, could be linked to the incidence of stroke. Of the 2,006 participants examined, 98 experienced a stroke during the 13 years of follow-up studies. Folic acid levels showed an inverse relationship to the risk of stroke, even after taking other stroke risk factors into account, such as age, gender, history of heart disease, blood pressure, and smoking.[33]

Decades of scientific research had made the problem clear and irrefutable: high levels of homocysteine in the blood initiate injuries to the blood vessel walls that lead to many of the diseases affecting the cardiovascular system. But do these studies also contain a clear solution? Yes, treating high levels of homocysteine and lowering the risk of cardiovascular disease may be as easy as including extra servings of dark green leafy vegetables or supplementing with B-complex vitamins.

## HOMOCYSTEINE: WHAT IS NORMAL?

The average person has an extremely small amount of homocysteine circulating in the bloodstream. For every 1,000 molecules of cholesterol there is generally only one molecule of homocysteine. It is amazing that such a tiny amount of homocysteine can dramatically increase the risk of heart attack, stroke and peripheral artery disease.

Researchers are currently trying to establish safe levels of homocysteine. In general, it appears that the lower the homocysteine level, the better. Based on the conclusions of several recent studies, homocysteine levels of less than 6 micromoles per liter of blood is ideal. Amounts of 10 micromoles per liter of blood used to be considered normal, but this level is increasingly interpreted as risky. The risk increases with the level, and more than 13 micromoles per liter is considered very dangerous. There appears to be no danger from low homocysteine levels.

Although the evidence shows elevated homocysteine to be a risk factor for cardiovascular disease, screening tests are not generally requested by most physicians. However, they are available. If your medical facility does not currently perform homocysteine assessments, it should be able to have an associated facility run the test. An easier homocysteine test is currently being developed and should increase the number of patients screened for elevated homocysteine levels.

## HOMOCYSTEINE AS A MARKER FOR VITAMIN DEFICIENCIES

Even marginal intake of the B vitamins folic acid and vitamin B6 causes homocysteine concentrations to creep up. Some researchers suggest that testing homocysteine levels is a good indicator of vitamin deficiencies. In fact, it is not uncommon for blood tests to mistakenly indicate adequate B vitamin levels, while homocysteine tests and a beneficial response to vitamin supplementation reveal B vitamin deficiencies.

# FOLIC ACID:
# THE FIRST LINE OF
# DEFENSE

ALTHOUGH FOLIC ACID was one of the last vitamins to be discovered, it performs several necessary functions in the body. It contributes to the growth of new cells and the replacement of old cells; it helps synthesize the genetic molecules DNA and RNA; and assists in the transport of carbon building bricks to the "construction sites" of the body. For example, red blood cells have a short life, averaging only 120 days, and must be replaced on a regular basis for optimal health. When folic acid is in short supply, red blood cells are not replaced, resulting in a type of anemia.

Folic acid seems to be the single most important nutrient in protecting against homocysteine. It protects the body from unusually high homocysteine levels by assisting another enzyme in converting homocysteine back to the amino acid methionine. If the body does not have adequate amounts of folic acid, homocysteine begins to accumulate. As levels of homocysteine rise, blood vessels are injured, arteriosclerosis accelerates and the risk of heart attack and stroke escalates. Low levels of folic acid are implicated in up to 40 percent of heart attacks and strokes, while increased folic acid intake could prevent as many as 56,000 deaths from cardiovascular disease.[34]

The evidence from scientific studies strongly supports folic acid's ability to lower homocysteine levels. The following excerpts from such studies reflect the growing consensus among cardiovascular disease researchers.

•Lars E. Brattstroøm, M.D., at University Hospital in Lund, Sweden writes "... folic acid therapy might well be of practical use in reducing plasma homocysteine."[35]

•Dr. Johan B. Ubbink, Faculty of Medicine, University of Pretoria, South Africa asserts that a daily B vitamin supplement that includes folic acid "may be both efficient and cost-effective to control elevated plasma homocysteine concentrations."[36]

•"[H]igh dose folic acid therapy almost invariably seems to reduce elevated plasma homocysteine concentrations in patients with renal or vascular disease and even decreases normal plasma homocysteine concentrations in normal non-folate deficient subjects," concludes G. Landgren in a recent article in the *Journal of Internal Medicine.*[37]

---

### Food Sources of Folic Acid

The name folic acid was derived from the same root word as foliage, so it is not surprising that some of the best dietary sources of this nutrient are dark green leafy vegetables.

| Food | Folic Acid (mcg) |
|---|---|
| Brewer's yeast (1 tablespoon) | 313 |
| Orange juice (1 cup) | 136 |
| Spinach (raw, 1 cup) | 106 |
| Romaine lettuce (1 cup) | 98 |
| Spinach (cooked, 1/2 cup) | 82 |
| Broccoli (cooked, 1/2 cup) | 38 |

---

## FOLIC ACID DEFICIENCY AND SAFETY

The Recommended Dietary Allowance (RDA) for folic acid was drastically reduced in 1989. Many physicians and researchers, in light of the recent links between folic acid, birth defects, and cardiovascular diseases, have urged going back to the previous, higher RDA. One prominent organization, the U.S. Public Health Service, now recommends a daily intake of 400 mcg of folic acid for all women—puberty through menopause—to prevent birth defects in their offspring. This recommendation is probably suitable for anyone wanting to reduce their homocysteine levels, and risk of heart attack or stroke.

Folic acid requirements increase in several situations, such as during pregnancy and lactation, during illness, and with the use of some drugs (including oral contraceptives, several cancer treatments, and alcohol). In addition, smokers have lower folic acid levels than nonsmokers and may require a higher intake to maintain normal status of this important B vitamin.

Deficiencies of folic acid are among the most common of all vitamin deficiencies. Symptoms, besides increased risk of birth defects and cardiovascular diseases, include anemia, irritability, weakness, weight loss, headaches, forgetfulness, and diarrhea.

Some researchers have called for widespread fortification of foods with folic acid as a sensible way to increase intake and protect against folic acid deficiency. Currently, the average folic acid intake is 242 mcg daily, far below the 400 mcg necessary to help prevent birth defects and elevated homocysteine levels. In fact, on any given day, only one out of two Americans meet their folic acid requirement. Since the bioavailability of folic acid from foods is 50 percent less than that of supplements and fortified foods, it seems appropriate to consider fortifying grains with folic acid as a way to protect the public.[38]

Indeed, starting in 1998, the FDA will require food makers to add folic acid to flour. Unfortunately, many doctors, including Harvard's Stampfer and Rimm, believe such food fortification will have limited benefits. Eating more leafy green vegetables, rich in folic acid, or taking supplements are preferable.

Folic acid is an extremely safe vitamin, and doses up to 1,000 times the RDA can be consumed without toxic effects. However, very large doses of folic acid may interfere with the bioavailability of zinc, and pregnant women on such dosages should consider a concurrent zinc supplement. As with any supplement during pregnancy, use only with your physician's knowledge and consent. Extreme caution should be used by epileptics supplementing with folic acid. Some evidence shows that this B vitamin may increase seizures.[39]

The main criticism of folic acid supplements or food fortification plans is that folic acid can "mask" a disease of vitamin B12 deficiency known as pernicious anemia. Left untreated, this anemia can result in severe neurological degeneration and even death. But this concern has little validity today.

Years ago, vitamin B12 deficiency was typically diagnosed by looking at red-blood cell abnormalities under a microscope. Very high doses of folic acid can mask these blood anomalies, allowing neurological damage from B12 deficiency to continue unnoticed. Today, a laboratory test for methylmalonic acid serves as a more sensitive and specific test for vitamin B12 deficiency, just as homocysteine is a highly sensitive test for folic acid deficiency.

Furthermore, the American Medical Association has, in a manner of speaking, blessed the relative safety of folic acid. In the AMA's *Archives of Internal Medicine,* Norman R.C. Campbell, M.D., wrote that folic acid is "unlikely to cause adverse effects" at daily doses up to 5,000 mcg (5mg.).[40] On average, 400-800 mcg (less than 1 mg) is sufficient for controling homocysteine in most people.

In the 1980s, Carlton Fredericks, Ph.D. suggested a simple safeguard for anyone contemplating folic acid supplements: take some vitamin B12 as well. Writing in *JAMA*, Dr. Boushey echoed this advice by suggesting that people take 1 mg of B12 with every 400 mcg tablet of folic acid. It's a simple solution. And by choosing a B-complex supplement, which includes folic acid, vitamin B12, and other B vitamins, or eating a variety of B vitamin-rich foods, there should be no risk of a masked case of pernicious anemia.

## HOMOCYSTEINE, FOLIC ACID, AND BIRTH DEFECTS

An adequate supply of folic acid is absolutely essential during the rapid growth and development of pregnancy. Inadequate folic acid in the early stages of pregnancy, often before a woman even knows she is pregnant, increases the risk of bearing a child with a neural tube defect (NTD), such as spina bifida or anencephaly, conditions where the embryonic neural tube that forms the future brain and spinal column fails to close properly.

The British Medical Research Council, in 1991, provided the landmark evidence that folic acid supplements prevent the recurrence of NTDs in women who already had an NTD-afflicted child. The following year, Andrew E. Czeizel, M.D., of Hungary showed that folic acid also prevented NTDs in women who had no history of NTD pregnancies. Numerous subsequent studies confirm that folic acid plays a major role in healthy pregnancies, reducing the risk of NTDs by up to 60 percent. Several other birth defects, including cleft lip, cleft palate, cardiovascular disorders, and impaired neurological development in newborns have also been linked to low maternal folic acid intake.

By some estimates, six pregnancies with NTDs occur

every single day and could be prevented by adequate folic acid intake. Although several health organizations agree that all women of childbearing age should consume at least 400 mcg of folic acid daily to prevent these birth defects, a recent poll finds that only 15 percent of women are aware of this recommendation and only 20 percent of women use a supplement that includes folic acid prior to their pregnancy. Adequate folic acid status is critical in the early weeks of a pregnancy, when the neural tube is forming. Although it is possible to consume this level of folic acid from the diet alone, it is difficult. Consequently, a multiple one-a-day type supplement that includes folic acid is the easiest way for most people to maintain adequate folic acid status.

Dr. James L. Mills at the National Institutes of Health in Bethesda, Maryland tested homocysteine levels in the mothers of 323 normal children and 81 infants born with an NTD and found that homocysteine levels are significantly higher in the mothers of children with birth defects. This suggests that homocysteine levels can be used as a risk marker of potential NTD pregnancies. The results of this study and another by researchers at the Trinity College, in Dublin, Ireland suggest that folic acid and vitamin B12 are important for reducing both homocysteine levels and the risk of neural tube birth defects during pregnancy.[35,36]

## FOLIC ACID DEFICIENCY, DNA DAMAGE AND CANCER

Folic acid also plays an essential role in a minute but profound process that chemists call "methylation." When methylation goes awry, it can damage your genes and set the stage for cancer, the second leading cause of death in the United States.

Quite simply, methylation entails the creation of molecules containing one atom of carbon and three atoms of hydrogen. These compounds are called methyl groups, and chemists write them out as $CH_3$. The body needs these methyl groups to make deoxyribonucleic acid (DNA), which forms your genes and chromosomes; ribonucleic acid (RNA), which translates DNA's code into proteins; and numerous other important substances, including adrenaline, serotonin, carnitine and creatine.

This may be far more biochemistry than you're interested in, but the important point to remember is that folic acid, choline and methionine are "methyl donors," meaning they donate $CH_3$ molecules to the methylation process. How important is this? Your DNA, created through methylation , is your body's equivalent of computer code. It programs everything from your eye color and height to your risk for cancer and other diseases. When your DNA functions normally, it tells each of your body's 60 trillion cells when and how to grow and when to, stop. Problems occur when DNA becomes damaged and gives cells incorrect instructions, such as to keep growing. In fact, studies have shown that deficiencies of methyl donors interfere with methylation and increase the risk of DNA damage and cancer.

In one recent study, Australian researchers studied 64 apparently healthy men,ages 50-70. Twenty-three percent of the men had low blood levels of folic acid, and 37 percent had moderately high levels of homocysteine. More than half of the men (56 percent) had abnormal blood levels of folic acid, vitamin B12, or homocysteine. Men with low levels of vitamins or high levels of homocysteine were much more likely to also have breaks in their DNA (measured in their white blood cells). Especially significant was the finding that men with elevated homocysteine levels, but apparently normal folic acid levels, were more likely to suffer from DNA breaks.[43]

Folic acid appears to prevent cancer in other ways as well. Bruce N. Ames, Ph.D., a professor at the University of California, Berkeley, and one of the world's leading molecular biologists, recently investigated exactly what happens to DNA when folic acid levels are inadequate. Normally, thymine is one of four proteins that make up DNA. When there isn't enough thymine, however, uracil (another protein) is incorrectly substituted. When normal DNA repair mechanisms remove excess uracil, they leave breaks in the DNA.

When breaks occur in one of DNA's two strands, they can often be repaired. Double-strand breaks are much more difficult to repair and therefore more dangerous, according to Ames. Because so much uracil accumulates during folic acid deficiency, the risk of double-strand breaks is especially greater. In a recent study of DNA breaks in people, Ames and his colleagues found that folic acid supplements dramatically decreased the amount of uracil being incorporated into DNA, "suggesting that, in folate-deficient people, increased folate intake may decrease the risk of many types of cancer.[44]

Low levels of folic acid have been implicated in the increased risk of several cancers, including colon, lung, and cervical cancer. Women who consume diets low in folic acid are at an increased risk for developing cervical dysplasia and cancer of the cervix, whereas optimal folic acid intake appears to prevent this precancerous condition. Gregorios Paspatis, M.D., at the Metaxa Cancer Hospital in Piraeus, Greece, has reported that low levels of folic acid increase the risk of colon adenoma, a type of colon tumor. Folic acid deficiency causes cellular damage that resembles the initial stages of cancer whereas optimal folic acid status may prevent the transformation of abnormal cells into cancerous cells.[45, 46, 47]

Folic acid may also protect against prostate cancer.

Richard S. Rivlin, M.D., of Memorial Sloan-Kettering Cancer Center, New York, reported at a scientific meeting that a new test, called the Prostate Specific Membrane Antigen (PSMA) will soon replace Prostate Specific Antigen (PSA) test for prostate cancer. The PSMA test measures the enzyme folate hydrolsae, Rivlin said that it implies that folic acid deficiency is involved in prostate cancer.[48]

Folic acid might protect against cancer by promoting normal activity of an anticancer gene. Young-In Kim, M.D., of the University of Toronto, Canada, recently investigated how folic acid deficiency specifically affected the p53 tumor-suppressor gene. Scientists believe that defects in this one gene may be the cause of more than 50 percent of all human cancers.

Kim discovered that a lack of folic acid resulted in DNA strand breaks in the p53 gene and also interfered with the methylation of DNA. These alterations to the p53 gene would likely increase the risk of cancer, Kim wrote in the *American Journal of Clinical Nutrition.*[49]

## FOLIC ACID, DEPRESSION AND ALZHEIMER'S DISEASE

Low levels of folic acid can impair mental performance. Maurizio Fava, M.D., of Massachusetts General Hospital, Boston, has reported that patients with low folic acid levels are more likely to suffer from melancholic (very severe) depression and are less likely to respond to antidepressent drug therapy. [50] In another study, Dutch researchers reported that patients with Alzheimer's disease had much higher levels of homocysteine than did other types of hospitalized patients and healthy subjects.[51]

In an article in the *Proceedings of the National Academy of*

*Sciences of the USA*, Bruce N. Ames, Ph.D., noted that DNA breaks caused by folic acid deficiency can impair mental function. Even moderately low levels of folic acid and vitamin B12 can affect thinking processes. The effect may be compounded by inadequate intake of antioxidant vitamins, such as vitamins C and E. Ames's findings support the important role of folic acid in preventing neurodegeneration.[52]

## SPECIAL CONSIDERATIONS FOR DIALYSIS PATIENTS

Kidney dialysis patients have much higher than average homocysteine levels, which contribute to their increased risk of cardiovascular diseases. M. Arnadottir, M.D., of the University Hospital in Lund, Sweden, found that four months of daily treatment with 5 mg of folic acid in 18 dialysis patients lowered homocysteine levels by 30 percent, which should translate into an improved cardiovascular risk profile.[53] "Supplementation of folic acid...may represent an innocuous yet effective means of reducing homocysteine that may reduce the occurrence of [cardiovascular disease] in patients undergoing dialysis," concludes Joy A. Riedman, M.S., Tufts University Schools of Medicine and Nutrition, in her review study.[54]

# "B" HEALTHY: VITAMIN B6, VITAMIN B12, CHOLINE, AND BETAINE

HIGH LEVELS OF HOMOCYSTEINE damage blood vessels and contribute to several cardiovascular diseases, including heart attacks, strokes, and peripheral artery disease. According to Manuel Rene Malinow, M.D., of Oregon Health Sciences University, Portland, the solution is just as clear as the problem. In an editorial published in the prestigious journal *Circulation* in June 1990, he wrote that "treatment of elevated levels of [homocysteine] is simple and innocuous...in most adult patients, small doses of folate (1-5 mg/day) are usually effective in rapidly reducing elevated levels..." Malinow explained that if a patient does not respond to the folic acid supplements, other supplements, such as vitamin B6, vitamin B12, choline, or betaine, almost always lower the resistant homocysteine levels.

## VITAMIN B6 FOR A HEALTHY HEART

As McCully clearly demonstrated, vitamin B6 (pyridoxine) is another one of the B vitamins essential for the complete breakdown and metabolism of the amino acid methionine. Low levels of vitamin B6 allow homocysteine levels to increase and initiate the atherosclerotic process. Unfortunately, low levels of vitamin B6 appear to be the rule rather than the exception in the U.S. population.

A study, published in the *American Journal of Clinical*

*Nutrition,* found that one-third of elderly, low-income people are deficient in vitamin B6. Malina Manore, Ph.D., of Arizona State University in Tempe, Arizona, noted that the two major causes of vitamin B6 deficiency are 1) inadequate intake of food sources of the vitamin, and 2) the presence of health problems, such as smoking, kidney disorders, diabetes, and heart disease, which interfere with vitamin B6 absorption and use.

Another study, analyzing a series of menus developed by health professionals, found that half of the menus failed to meet the RDA for vitamin B6, suggesting that the general public probably has difficulty designing and eating meals that meet vitamin B6 requirements. The elderly, individuals with malabsorption disorders, women on oral contraceptives, alcoholics, and anyone with a poor diet are at risk for compromised vitamin B6 status.

A unique situation in Texas provided McCully with a special opportunity to examine the heart protection of vitamin B6. Over the past three decdes, citizens of Titus County, Texas have been encouraged to take B6 supplements (by the news media and by simple word of mouth) to prevent a wide range of health conditions, including carpal tunnel syndrome, rhuematic disease, diabetes, and heart disease. [55] On average, the people living in this county consume twice the Recommended Dietary Allowance (RDA) for B6.

Afetr tracking heart disease deaths in this county, McCully, along with John M. Ellis, M.D., of Titus County Memorial Hospital, found that individuals who regularly took vitamin B6 supplements (for as little as one year and up to 17 years) slashed their risk of heart attack by 73 percent. While non-supplementers who developed heart disease experienced their first heart attack at approximately age 59, B6 users with heart disease postponed their first heart attack until the ripe old age of 75. And of those who died of a heart attack, the B6 users lived an average of eight extra years, compared to those not taking vitamin B6 supplements. Clearly, B6 (even without the other B vitamins) is a powerful way to reduce homocysteine levels and the risk of heart attack.

Even if you already know you have coronary artery disease, homocysteine levels are still important. Norwegian researchers, after recording homocysteine levels of 587 heart disease patients and tracking their health for almost five years, report that "...homocysteine levels are a strong predictor of mortality..."[56] This means that even for people with heart disease, having high homocysteine levels makes it more likely that you will die from a heart attack, while low homocysteine levels make it more likely that you will survive.

## VITAMIN B6 BASICS

Vitamin B6 is involved in the metabolism of proteins and carbohydrates. Symptoms of vitamin B6 deficiency are vague, but include weakness, mental confusion, elevated homocysteine levels, anemia, and insomnia. Oral contraceptives increase vitamin B6 requirements. The RDA for vitamin B6 is 2 mg and 1.6 mg daily for adult men and women, respectively.

Good food sources of vitamin B6 include beans, nuts, bananas, cabbage, cauliflower, potatoes, and whole-grain cereals and breads. Foods made with white flour are poor sources of the vitamin because "enrichment" does not replace the vitamin B6 lost in the refining of whole grains. Meat also provides vitamin B6, but not enough to offset its methionine.

Although negative reactions to vitamin B6 are rare, there is a potential for toxicity. Long-term supplemental intake of 500 mg (250 times higher than the RDA) or more may cause permanent nervous system damage. However, supplements providing RDA levels or even up to 10-50 mg of vitamin B6 are generally safe.

Vitamin B6 supplements have been used with some success in treating asthma, insomnia, carpal tunnel syndrome, premenstrual syndrome, and to improve immunity.

### Good Food Sources of Vitamin B6

| Food | Vitamin B6 (mg) |
|---|---|
| Banana (1 medium) | 0.89 |
| Salmon (3 ounces) | 0.63 |
| Chicken (3 ounces) | 0.51 |
| Halibut (3 ounces) | 0.39 |
| Hamburger (3 ounces) | 0.39 |
| Tuna (canned, 3 ounces) | 0.36 |
| Broccoli (1 medium stalk) | 0.35 |
| Potato (1 medium) | 0.20 |

Note: While meat is a good source of vitamin B6, it provides still more methionine, which leads to higher homocysteine levels. The B6 in meat alone is inadequate for properly metabolizing methionine and homocysteine.

## ESKIMO AND VEGETARIAN DIETS

The ratio of vitamin B6 to protein intake may have more to do with vitamin B6 status and health than the intake of the vitamin per se. Researchers have puzzled over why both vegetarians and traditional meat-and-fat-eating Eskimos have a lower risk of cardiovascular disease than does the typical American. A traditional Eskimo diet provides more protein and fat and less vitamin B6 than typical American or vegetarian diets, yet this population group rarely suffers from cardiovascular disease. The answer to this apparent contradiction may be found in cooking methods. Heating and cooking food, a common procedure in American kitchens, destroys most of its vitamin B6. Eskimos, by eating many of their foods raw, preserve vitamin levels.

The lesson to be learned from the Eskimo diet example is not that Americans should start consuming large amounts of raw meat, but rather that cardiovascular disease is not inevitable. A key to preventing heart attacks and strokes includes maintaining optimal status of the B vitamins. In particular, vitamin B6 seems to clear homocysteine out of the blood.

In a slightly different way, vegetarian diets reduce the risk, and may even treat, many cardiovascular diseases. First, limiting or removing meat from the diet tends to reduce intake of saturated fat and cholesterol, which lowers blood cholesterol levels and the risk of arteriosclerosis. Second, eating very little meat also tends to reduce protein intake, which would improve the ratio of the amino acid methionine to vitamin B6 in the diet, which lowers homocysteine levels. Finally, the meat that is removed from the diet is often replaced with grains, fruits, and vegetables. Many of these foods, which are rich in fiber, vitamins, and minerals and low in fat, also reduce homocysteine and cholesterol levels.

A vegetarian diet provides a large amount of vitamin B6 relative to protein. In addition, intake of the amino acid methionine (the source of homocysteine) is low, resulting in lower levels of homocysteine and lower risk of cardiovascular disease. "The use of a low methionine vegetarian diet has been proposed as a new approach to preventing arteriosclerosis," according to McCully.

All in all, the evidence strongly supports the role of vitamin B6 in reducing homocysteine, and in turn, the risk of heart attack, stroke, and peripheral artery disease. One study found that vitamin B6 supplements in mildly hyperhomocysteinemic patients diagnosed with cardiovascular diseases significantly reduced homocysteine levels in 56 percent of the patients. Michiel van den Berg, M.D., Department of Surgery, Institute for Cardiovascular Research, Free University Hospital in The Netherlands has found that a combined treatment of vitamin B6 and folic acid "...normalizes homocysteine metabolism in virtually all patients..."[57]

## WOMEN, B VITAMINS, AND CARDIOVASCULAR DISEASE

The only time most women think about cardiovascular disease is when worrying about the health of their husbands or other male family members. Unfortunately, most women should give more thought to their own risk of cardiovascular disease. The latest studies show that one out of every nine women between the ages of 45 and 64 has some type of cardiovascular disease. In fact, heart attacks are the number one killer of American women, surpassing mortality from breast cancer and other diseases.

Still, women have been almost completely ignored in the majority of cardiovascular disease research studies. While it is true that heart attacks occur more frequently in men, the heart attacks that women do have are more likely to be fatal. The gender difference in cardiovascular disease comes down to when each gender is at the greatest risk of disease, rather than which gender is at risk. The greatest risk for heart attacks in men generally peaks a full decade before the risk for women peaks—in the years after menopause.

Premenopausal women are at the lowest risk for developing atherosclerosis, heart attacks, or other cardiovascular diseases. However, cardiovascular disease risks do rise alarmingly when these women use oral contraceptives. Some studies indicate that the hormones in the oral contraceptives increase the conversion of methionine into homocysteine. This process is very similar to that found in individuals with certain enzyme deficiencies.

Another confounding factor is the prevalence of vitamin deficiencies, particularly of vitamin B6 and folic acid among oral contraceptive users. Since these vitamins are needed to neutralize homocysteine, inadequate levels of B vitamins lead to a dangerous accumulation of homocysteine in the bloodstream among women who use birth control pills. Atherosclerosis has been reported in women with a history of oral contraceptive use, and the type of blood vessel damage is very similar to that seen in people with documented cases of homocysteinemia. According to McCully, it seems prudent for any women currently using oral contraceptives to eat extra servings of foods rich in the B vitamins, especially vitamin B6 and folic acid, or to choose a supplement containing these important nutrients.

## VITAMIN B12: ANOTHER IMPORTANT VITAMIN

Vitamin B12 is also essential during the metabolism of protein, fat, and carbohydrates. As with folic acid and vitamin B6, vitamin B12 must be present to rid the body of harmful amounts of homocysteine.

The deficiency disease most associated with vitamin B12 is pernicious (or megaloblastic) anemia. This anemia can result from a low intake of vitamin B12 or inadequate gastric secretion of "intrinsic factor," a substance necessary for vitamin B12 absorption. Vitamin B12 is stored in the body and deficiency symptoms do not develop for several years after poor intake or impaired absorption. Pernicious anemia, as with other anemias, seriously interferes with the body's production of red blood cells and results in fatigue and poor concentration.

Other symptoms of vitamin B12 deficiency, in addition to pernicious anemia and elevated homocysteine, include disorientation, numbness, confusion, agitation, dizziness, hallucinations, impaired immunity, nausea, and vomiting.

Vitamin B12 deficiencies are more common in people during mid- to late life and in strict vegetarians (who exclude all animal products). As many as 15 percent of the elderly may have vitamin B12 deficiencies. Restoring optimal vitamin B12 status may improve mood, cognitive function, and even symptoms of Alzheimer's disease in older populations. Hans J. Naurath, M.D., Department of Geriatric Medicine, University Witten-Heddecke, Germany, recommends testing homocysteine levels as the most precise way to identify vitamin B12 deficiencies, especially in the vulnerable elderly populations.[58]

---

### Food Sources of Vitamin B12

Vitamin B12 is only found in foods of animal origin, such as meat, fish, and dairy products. The vitamin B12 requirement for adults is 2 mcg daily. There is very little, if any, risk of toxicity, even at very large intakes of this vitamin.

| Food | Vitamin B12 (mcg) |
|---|---|
| Beef liver (3 ounces) | 93.0 |
| Beef (3 ounces) | 2.0 |
| Tuna (canned, 3 ounces) | 1.8 |
| Yogurt (1 cup) | 1.5 |
| Milk (1 cup) | 0.9 |
| Chicken (3 ounces) | 0.4 |
| Cheddar cheese (1 ounce) | 0.2 |

---

Men with moderately high levels of homocysteine have significantly lower vitamin B12 levels, and supplements of vitamin B12 alone have been shown to lower their homocysteine concentrations.[59, 60] However, vitamin B12 is not usually used by itself to treat high levels of homocysteine, but rather as part of a B-complex supplement. A combined supplement plan provides the benefits of all the B vitamins, improves the homocysteine-lowering response, and prevents secondary or masked deficiencies.

Nitrous oxide (laughing gas) is often used as an anesthetic during surgery. It can destroy vitamin B12 and cause symptoms of nerve damage. Doctors reported one case in which a 70-year-old woman was given anesthesia for 105 minutes during surgery. Ten days later, she developed a general sense of weakness and leg pains, and four weeks later could not walk and suffered sharp pain when touched lightly on the legs. When tested, her blood B12 levels were a fraction of normal. After receiving B12 injections, she improved. This is one more, though little recognized, surgical stress that can hinder the recovery of patients.[61]

## VITAMIN B12 AND DIABETES

The risk of developing a cardiovascular disease is much higher in diabetics. Atsushi Araki, M.D., of the Tokyo Metropolitan Geriatric Hospital found that diabetic patients with signs of "macroangiopathy"—coronary or cerebral artery disease—had higher levels of homocysteine than other diabetic patients or healthy individuals. Treatment with vitamin B12 significantly decreased their homocysteine levels. "The findings on the association between elevated plasma homocysteine and atherosclerotic disease in diabetic patients are consistent with other reports on the relationship between plasma homocysteine levels and cerebrovascular disease in nondiabetic subjects," wrote Araki.[62]

# THE CHOLINE CONNECTION

Choline is a vitamin B-like substance that is not technically classified as an official vitamin because the body can produce it. However, choline is essential to health and it may soon be classified as an essential nutrient. For example, it is a building block for phospholipids, the fats needed in cell membranes. Choline also contributes to the production of the neurotransmitter acetylcholine, which is important in brain function and memory.

To produce choline, the body must have adequate amounts of folic acid. Often, deficiencies of folic acid and choline go hand in hand. Choline is found in foods as free choline or as part of the compound lecithin. Good food sources of choline include eggs, organ meats, lean meat, brewer's yeast, wheat germ, soybeans, and peanuts. There is no established requirement or toxicity levels for choline, but the average diet provides between 700 and 1,000 mg daily.

Choline was discovered early on to reduce homocysteine levels and the risk of cardiovascular diseases. As far back as 1938, when numerous experiments with cholesterol-rich diets in rabbits were performed, researchers reported that choline delayed and even prevented the development of atherosclerosis in rabbits fed these large amounts of cholesterol. McCully, the pioneering homocysteine researcher, later noted that choline deficiency raised homocysteine levels by altering the metabolism of the amino acid methionine, with the end result being "...accelerated vascular damage and arteriosclerotic lesions."

Aside from lowering homocysteine levels, choline has other health benefits. For instance, the brain contains high levels of choline, and researchers at Harvard Consolidated Department of Psychiatry in Boston suggest that dwindling brain choline levels in aging adults may be an underlying factor for age-related psychiatric illnesses, such as depression and Alzheimer's disease.[63] Another group of Harvard researchers suggests, in a study of six patients with manic depression, that choline supplements of 3-8 grams daily (combined with lithium medication) improve the effectiveness of treatment for this mental disorder. [64]

## THE BENEFITS OF BETAINE

Betaine is another beneficial substance found in some foods and supplements, and produced by the body. Like the B vitamins, large supplemental doses of betaine limit the unhealthy buildup of homocysteine. While betaine is not usually the first choice in treating elevated homocysteine levels, it often plays an important role in difficult-to-treat cases. Several studies have reported that betaine supplements successfully lower homocysteine in cases in which vitamin B6 and folic acid failed.[65, 66]

Betaine supplements used to lower homocysteine levels are sometimes confused with a digestive aid called betaine HCI. In the case of betaine HCI, the betaine molecule is merely acting as a delivery system for the HCI (hydrochloric acis), which is taken to acidify the stomach and improve the digestive process. However, when betaine is used to lower homocysteine levels, the reverse is true; the HCI has no effect and the betaine is the active part of the supplement. For this reason, supplements of betaine without the HCI attached to it would be more desirable for individuals with high homocysteine levels. However, betaine plays a minor role in controlling homocysteine, and so it is much better to emphasize the B vitamins than this nutrient.

# RECOMMENDATIONS FOR A HEALTHY CARDIOVASCULAR SYSTEM

EVERY 34 SECONDS, a cardiovascular disease takes the life of an American. Almost 5 million years of potential life are lost yearly (based on a 75-year lifespan) because of premature deaths from heart attacks, strokes, and other cardiovascular diseases. Something must be done to turn this deadly tide of deaths and shortened lives.

Scientists, physicians, and patients have made some progress. In one ten-year period, 1981 to 1991, death rates from all forms of cardiovascular diseases declined by about 25 percent. But so much more remains to be done for the estimated 56 million Americans who currently have a cardiovascular disease.

After decades of being disregarded by the scientific community, homocysteine is finally being acknowledged as a major risk factor for heart attack, stroke, and peripheral artery disease. In a recent interview, Carol J. Boushey, Ph.D., a prominent homocysteine researcher, said, "Think where cholesterol was 20 years ago—it was just beginning to be considered an important agent in cardiovascular disease. Homocysteine, today, is in the same place."

Scientists know that homocysteine levels increase with age. It is not coincidental that B vitamin deficiencies are also prevalent among the elderly. Dangerously high homocysteine concentrations can be found in up to 40 percent of older adults, which triples their risk of a heart attack and doubles the incidence of hardening of the carotid arteries—one the leading causes of stroke.

And now for the good news. Scientists have found a simple and effective method for lowering homocysteine levels. This surprisingly easy, cheap, and painless answer is found through supplementing the diet with a B-complex supplement containing folic acid, B6, B12, choline, and perhaps betaine.

## THE BIGGER PICTURE

The long-running Framingham Heart Study identified the primary risk factors of cardiovascular disease as high blood pressure, cigarette smoking, and high blood levels of cholesterol (especially elevated LDL cholesterol). Secondary risk factors include obesity, diabetes, stress, physical inactivity, family history, male gender, and increasing age. Today, new research from the Framingham Heart Study confirms that homocysteine should be added to this list of cardiovascular disease risk factors. In fact, individuals suffering from cardiovascular disease have been found to have 30 percent higher homocysteine concentrations than their healthy counterparts.

Homocysteine and blood cholesterol both contribute to arteriosclerosis, the underlying cause of most heart attacks. However, homocysteine may lay the groundwork for cholesterol to do its damage. Some evidence indicates that homocysteine attacks and strips away surface cells on the blood vessel walls. These bare patches are often filled in with other cell types. Cholesterol is attracted to these growing diseased patches, called atheromas. Atheromas then block the flow of blood and injure passing blood cells, causing them to clot, setting the stage for a heart attack or stroke. While homocysteine may be more damaging to blood vessels than cholesterol, it is easier to correct by increasing the intake of B vitamins.

## PUTTING IT INTO PRACTICE

Heart disease is not an inevitable effect of aging. Although it is true that cardiovascular diseases are more likely as we age, heart disease does not have to be a foregone conclusion. In some countries, atherosclerosis and other forms of cardiovascular disease are virtually unheard of, even in the elderly. It is very telling, however, that when people from such countries move to Western countries and change to our diet, their cardiovascular disease risk soon rises to match ours. The opposite, however, is also true. If we modify our Western diet to be more like the typical diets of countries with a low risk of heart disease, our cardiovascular systems may well become more resistant to heart disease.

The countries with the healthiest cardiovascular systems are spread out around the globe—from the Mediterranean to Asia—but the typical diets of these countries have several key elements in common. Nutritionists have determined many of these universal dietary factors which protect the cardiovascular system. Seven of these heart-saving nutrition secrets are:

1) Cut down on dietary fat.
2) Bulk up on fiber.
3) Choose antioxidant-rich fruits and vegetables.
4) Consume plenty of B vitamins.
5) Include servings of fish.
6) Incorporate garlic.
7) Add in soy foods.

Although controlling your homocysteine levels with B vitamins is of paramount importance, you can do other things to further shore up your defenses against heart disease and stroke. Let's take a closer look at each of these healthy diet tips.

### 1) Cut down on dietary fat.

Eating a low-fat diet is among the most important dietary weapons for lowering your risk of heart disease. Aside from reducing the overall fat intake of the diet, there are certain types of fat which are more dangerous, in terms of heart disease, than others. Unquestionably, the biggest offender of the fat family is saturated fat. Diets high in saturated fat are ominously linked to a skyrocketing risk of cardiovascular disease (as well as other health problems).[67] The most common sources of saturated fat are beef, pork, poultry, eggs, dairy products (milk, cheese, ice cream, and others), coconut, and palm oil. Meanwhile, people who avoid saturated fat have a lower risk of developing heart disease, and if they already have heart disease, their symptoms may actually regress if they switch to a low-fat diet.

The connection between fat and heart disease probably is at least part of the reason vegetarians—who tend to have low-fat diets—are less likely to die from heart disease.[68] An extreme vegetarian diet (containing no meat, dairy, or eggs), especially when combined with exercise and stress management skills, may even reverse heart disease.[69, 70]

Another type of fat, trans-fatty acids—found in margarine and other processed foods containing "hydrogenated" oils—is linked to an increased risk of heart disease.[71] The typical Western diet is loaded with processed foods, and consequently Americans consume more than 600 million pounds of trans-fatty acids each year. Individually, trans-fatty acids account for up to 12 percent of the total fat intake of an average American. The heart disease risk triggered by trans-fatty acids is serious business indeed. By some estimates, people who eat large amounts of trans-fatty acids increase their risk of heart disease by a whopping 27 percent. Consequently, margarine and other foods containing partially hydrogenated oils should be avoided whenever possible.

*2) Bulk up on fiber.*

Fat and fiber often act like a seesaw in the diet. As one is deemphasized, the other tends to become more of a focus. For a healthy heart, eating less fat and more fiber is the way to go. There are two types of fiber: soluble and insoluble. The soluble fibers in such foods as oat bran, fruits, some vegetables, and beans have been shown to lower cholesterol levels and thereby reduce the risk of heart disease.[72, 73] Insoluble fiber, although not implicated in reducing the risk of heart disease, has other health benefits. It simply makes sense to eat more of all types of fiber.

*3) Choose antioxidant-rich fruits and vegetables.*

As mentioned earlier in this book, free radical damage to LDL cholesterol amplifies the potential of LDL to damage blood vessels and initiate cardiovascular disease. Antioxidants, such as vitamin E, vitamin C, and the carotenoids, shield LDL cholesterol from free radical damage, which in turn lowers the risk of heart disease. [74, 75, 76]

Of the antioxidants, vitamin E is truly a nutritional star when it comes to heart disease. But don't take our word for it. Instead, you can take the word of such esteemed researchers as those from Harvard Medical School. After tracking the health and supplement use of 125,000 male and female health professionals for up to eight years, they found that individuals who took vitamin E supplements (of 100 IU or more daily for two years) were 40 percent less likely to develop heart disease.[77, 78] And this study is just the tip of the iceberg when it comes to vitamin E. The Cambridge Heart Antioxidant Study (CHAOS) also found vitamin E beneficial for the cardiovascular system. Supplementing with vitamin E (400 IU or 800 IU) for 17 months lowered the risk of heart attack by 77 percent in the 2,002 male and female study participants who were diagnosed with atherosclerosis and included in this study.[79]

Vitamin C is no slouch when it comes to protecting the heart and blood vessels. When vitamin C intakes are compared, people with the highest intake of vitamin C (generally those who supplement regularly) are the least likely to die from heart disease. In fact, mortality rates from cardiovascular disease are 45 percent lower in those with the highest vitamin C levels.[80]

Flavonoids, vitamin-like compounds found in many different foods, such as red wine, green tea, and many vegetables, are also powerful antioxidants which neutralize free radicals and strengthen the cardiovascular system. A series of studies involving middle-aged Dutch men reports that those with the highest intake of flavonoids (from tea, fruits, and vegetables) have a 73 percent lower risk of suffering a stroke than those with a low flavonoid intake.[81]

*4) Consume plenty of B vitamins.*

As discussed throughout this book, the B vitamins—folic acid, vitamin B6, and vitamin B12 in particular—are a powerful way to reduce the risk of cardiovascular diseases by clearing the dangerous substance homocysteine out of the blood.

## 5) Include servings of fish.

Dishing up fish shields the heart and blood vessels from heart disease, according to a large body of research. Although health experts are always praising the benefits of a low-fat diet, there's an exception to every rule, and with fat the exception is fish oil. Omega-3 fatty acids in the oil of cold-water fish (such as salmon, mackerel and tuna) benefit the cardiovascular system in several ways, such as by reducing total cholesterol and LDL-cholesterol levels, raising HDL-cholesterol levels and inhibiting the "clumping" of blood platelets that could otherwise initiate a heart attack or stroke. And it doesn't take much fish to provide protection. The amount of omega-3 fatty acids consumed in just one serving of fish per week can cut the risk of heart attack in half.[82]

## 6) Incorporate garlic.

Garlic is one of the oldest medicinal plants, and modern research confirms its amazing disease prevention and health promotion qualities, particularly for ensuring a healthy heart. Take, for example, a study of men at risk for heart disease who were given either garlic supplements or look-alike dummy pills.[83] Those taking the garlic supplements for six months showed significant reductions in their total cholesterol and LDL cholesterol levels, as well as lower blood pressure. Although you may run the risk of "garlic breath," your heart will thank you for dishing up plenty of garlicky cuisine.

## 7) Add soy foods.

One of the reasons soy foods, such as tofu and soy milk, may help prevent heart disease is that they take the place of some of the meat and dairy products in the diet. But soy has some heart-protecting properties—namely, the isoflavonoids— of its own. Research shows that soy dramatically lowers cholesterol levels. When 38 different soy studies were pooled together and reexamined, it was found that in 89 percent of the studies, soy slashed the cholesterol levels of the study participants.[84]

## CHECKLIST OF HEART-PROTECTING SUPPLEMENTS

Nutritional supplements can go a long way in helping you achieve the seven heart-saving nutrition secrets discussed above. According to nutrition experts, supplements of the following nutrients each day may be helpful additions to your personal heart disease prevention plan.

| Supplement: | How Much: |
| --- | --- |
| Vitamin E | 200 - 400 IU |
| Vitamin C | 1 - 2 grams |
| Flavonoids | 35 - 1,000 mg |
| Garlic | 600 - 900 mg |
| Soy | 20 - 30 grams |
| Fish oil (omega-3 fatty acids) | 3 grams |

## CHOOSING A HEALTHY LIFESTYLE

Keeping the cardiovascular system healthy takes more than just eating right; lifestyle choices also play an important role in determining who will, or won't, develop heart disease. Topping this list of lifestyle factors is smoking. There is little question that smoking is directly related to heart disease, as well as numerous other health problems.[85] There are no two ways about it: if you smoke, quit; and if you don't smoke, don't start. Quitting smoking will lessen the risk of having a heart attack, and after ten to 14 years of not smoking, an ex-smoker's risk of heart attack will functionally be that of a lifetime nonsmoker.[86]

The benefits of exercise for promoting overall health, as well as a healthy heart and blood vessels are also well known.[87] You don't have to be an Olympic athlete to benefit from physical activity. Even a regular regimen of walking can lower the likelihood that you will be stricken with heart disease.[88] Part of the benefit of regular exercise is probably related to weight loss, since exercisers are less likely to be obese, while obesity is—in itself—a risk factor for heart disease.[89] Even modest weight loss in overweight individuals, if it is maintained, can greatly improve cardiovascular health.[90]

"Type A" personalities—that is, overachievers who constantly feel highly stressed, time-conscious, impatient, competitive, and aggressive—are more likely than their more relaxed "Type B" counterparts to suffer from heart disease.[91, 92] On the other hand, reducing stress and feelings of hostility reduces the risk of heart disease.[93] There are many ways to cope more effectively with the inevitable stressors of life, including exercise, meditation, yoga, visualization, biofeedback and muscle relaxation.

## THE HOMOCYSTEINE REDUCTION PROGRAM

Cardiovascular diseases account for one out of every two deaths in the United States—you don't have to be one of them. Of course, heart disease is a complex disease, with a myriad of factors contributing to its development, yet homocysteine stands out as one of the strongest of these risk factors. By the most conservative of estimates, a high level of homocysteine in the blood directly accounts for one in every ten fatal cases of heart disease in men, and a slightly lower percentage in women.

It may seem amazing, but study after study presented in this book has demonstrated that a handful of simple and cheap nutrients—folic acid, vitamin B6, vitamin B12, choline, and betaine—reduce homocysteine levels, and thus the risk of heart disease. In fact, if everyone's folic acid intake was increased to 400 mcg daily in this country, several hundred thousand lives each year might be saved. Combined with the dietary and lifestyle advice given earlier in this chapter, it's clear that there are many ways in which you can lower your risk of heart disease.

Eat more foods rich in the homocysteine-fighting B vitamins—unfortunately, for most people, it's not as easy as it sounds. It is difficult to consume the optimal levels for these nutrients from food sources alone. For example, it takes 10 cups of broccoli or 11 bananas every day to consume the level of folic acid or vitamin B6 necessary to reduce elevated homocysteine levels. This isn't to say that choosing a combination of foods rich in the B vitamins isn't helpful. (Feel free to consult the tables of food sources of folic acid, vitamin B6, and vitamin B12 given earlier in the book and regularly include these foods in your diet) Pay particular attention to leafy green vegetables, such as spinach, and dark green vegetables, such as broccoli—these are "power" foods which support good health on a number of different levels, aside from lowering homocysteine.

---

## A Note to Physicians

Despite overwhelming evidence in the scientific literature, very few hospitals or medical centers test homocysteine as a risk marker for cardiovascular diseases. As we go to press, a new, easier test is being introduced. We encourage physicians and their patients to ask for and use this test in assessing homocysteine levels. By conservative estimates, more than 56,000 deaths every year could be prevented by identifying patients with high homocysteine levels and treating them with simple B vitamin supplements.

## THE BEST DEFENSE

Nutritional surveys confirm that deficiencies of the B vitamins are prevalent in the United States. In addition, research shows that if one B vitamin is missing from the diet, chances are good that most, if not all, of the others will also be in short supply. These widespread B vitamin deficiencies result in dangerously high homocysteine levels. However, since the majority of doctors do not assess homocysteine levels in their patients, the best offense to prevent cardiovascular diseases appears to be a good defense—supplementing with B vitamins.

All of the nutrients discussed in this book (i.e. folic acid, vitamin B6, vitamin B12, choline, and betaine) interrupt the production of homocysteine or help to quench its metabolism. Although each nutrient functions at a different stage, all lower the blood levels of homocysteine and reduce the risk of cardiovascular disease. Maintaining an optimal intake of these nutrients has the added benefit of preventing and treating other health disorders. For example, folic acid prevents birth defects and colon cancer, vitamin B6 may treat carpal tunnel syndrome and premenstrual syndrome, and vitamin B12 plays an important role in the nervous system.

If it is so easy to prevent tens of thousands of heart attacks, strokes, and cases of peripheral artery disease each year with vitamin supplements why isn't it being done? Unlike cholesterol-lowering or high blood pressure-lowering drugs, vitamin supplements do not have the backing of major drug companies. Drug companies spend millions of dollars in research and development, and must recoup that money from the sales of their drugs. Folic acid and the other B vitamins exist naturally in foods; they cannot be patented, and, therefore, are not aggressively marketed as major money-makers for the drug companies.

# THREE EASY STEPS TO LOWER HOMOCYSTEINE

*Step one: Include plentiful amounts of B vitamin-rich foods in your diet.*

Examples of folic acid-rich foods are orange juice, fortified breakfast cereal, spinach, broccoli, romaine lettuce and collard greens. Examples of foods high in vitamin B6 are banana, avocado, spinach and whole grains. (Although many meats are high in vitamin B6, their high levels of the amino acid methionine makes them undesirable for maintaining optimal homocysteine levels)

*Step two: Avoid foods which contribute to rising homocysteine levels.*

Certain foods can contribute to the body's homocysteine burden, and individuals concerned with their homocysteine levels may consider minimizing these foods in their diet. For instance, a high intake of the amino acid methionine leads to an increase in homocysteine levels. In general, most foods high in protein (especially animal-based foods) provide the body with methionine. Since Americans tend to consume far more protein than is required by the body, eating less protein (particularly protein from meat and dairy foods) may be beneficial.

Diets based on refined grains and those that include a lot of sugar can indirectly raise homocysteine levels. Refined carbohydrates, such as white flour and sugar, are depleted of B vitamins in their manufacturing process. Since the body requires B vitamins in the digestion of these foods, they can actually drain body stores of the B vitamins needed to keep homocysteine levels in check. Whole grains would be a better dietary choice.

*Step three: Supplement with homocysteine-fighting nutrients.*

Higher intakes of the nutrients folic acid, vitamin B6, vitamin B12, choline, and betaine are well researched for their ability (alone and in combination) to lower levels of homocysteine.

Those who find it difficult to incorporate ample amounts of the food sources of the B vitamins known to lower homocysteine levels should take supplements. Capsules or tablets of these B vitamins are a convenient (and inexpensive) option for anyone concerned with preventing or treating cardiovascular diseases. And to make it even easier, the following table shows—based on the latest research—the optimal intake levels of these nutrients you should look for in a dietary supplement.

The following supplemental amounts of nutrients have been used successfully, both separately or in combination, to lower homocysteine levels.

| Nutrient | Effective Intake Range |
|---|---|
| Folic Acid | 400 mcg - 2 mg |
| Vitamin B6 | 10 - 50 mg |
| Vitamin B12 | 400 - 1,000 mcg |
| Choline | 700 - 1,000 mg |
| Betaine | 250 - 3,000 mg |

A high-potency daily multiple-vitamin supplement should provide the basic amounts of the B vitamins needed to prevent homocysteine levels from rising to dangerous levels. Separate supplements of folic acid, vitamin B6, and vitamin B12 at higher doses may need to be taken to lower very high or resistant homocysteine levels. However, supplementing with all three vitamins, which will prevent possible imbalances from high doses of just one B vitamin, is often a good idea. In other words, start with a comprehensive multivitamin formula (which includes the B vitamins) or a B-complex supplement. You can add a separate folic acid supplement—start with 400 mcg. In very rare individuals, higher intakes of the homocysteine-fighting nutrients may be needed, but if this is the case, a physician should be consulted.

Although many of the causes and steps in the progression of cardiovascular diseases remain unclear to scientists, one thing is clear—the B vitamins lower homocysteine levels, which in turn can save tens of thousands of lives—and perhaps yours.

# NOTES

1. C. J. Boushey et al., "A quantitative assessment of plasma homocysteine as a risk factor for vascular disease," *JAMA*, October 4,1995; 274: 1049-1057.

2. J. B.Ubbink, "Vitamin B-12, vitamin B-6, and folate nutritional status in men with hyperhomocysteinemia," *American Journal of Clinical Nutrition*, January 1993;57:47-53.

3. J. Selhub et al., "Vitamin status and intake as primary determinants of homocysteinemia in an elderly population," *JAMA*, December 8, 1993, 270:2693-2698.

4. *Council for Responsible Nutrition News*, May 1995.

5. P. Frosst, et al., A candidate genetic risk factor for vascular disease: a common mutation in methylenetetrahydrofolate reductase," *Nature Genetics* 10 (May, 1995):111-3.

6. A. M. Molloy, et al., "Thermolabile variant of 5,10-methylenetetrahydrofolate reductase associated with low red-cell folates: implications for folate intake recommendations," *Lancet* 349 (May 31, 1997):1591-93.

7. M. J. Stampfer and E. B. Rimm "Folate and cardiovascular disease: Why we need a trial now," *Journal of the American Medical Association*, 275 (June 26, 1996):1829-30.

8. Ibid.

9. S. Parthasarathy, "Oxidation of low-density lipoprotein by thiol compounds leads to its recognition by the acetyl LDL receptor," *Biochimica et Biophysica Acta* 917 (1987): 337-40.

10. A. J. Olszewski et al., "Homocysteine metabolism and the oxidative modification of proteins and lipids," *Free Radical Biology & Medicine* 14 (1993): 683-93.

11. E. J. Schaefer et al., "Lipoprotein(a) levels and risk of coronary heart disease in men," *JAMA*, 271 (3) (6 April 1994): 999-1003.

12. J. B. Ubbink et al., "Results of B-vitamin supplementation study used in prediction model to define a reference range for plasma homocysteine," *Clinical Chemistry* 41 (7) (1995): 1033-37.

13. K. S. McCully, "Vascular pathology of homocysteinemia: Implications for the pathogenesis of arteriosclerosis," *American Journal of Pathology* 56 (1) (July 1969): 111-28.

14. K. S. McCully and R. B. Wilson, "Homocysteine theory of arteriosclerosis," *Atherosclerosis* 22 (1975): 215-27.

15. K. S. McCully, "Homocysteinemia and arteriosclerosis," *American Heart Journal* 83 (4) (April 1972): 571-73.

16. M. J. Stampfer et al., "A prospective study of plasma homocyst[e]ine and risk of myocardial infarction in US physicians," *JAMA* 268 (7) (August 1992): 877-81.

17. K. S. McCully, "Homocysteine thiolactone in arteriosclerosis and cancer," *Research Communications in Chemical Pathology & Pharmacology* 59 (1) (January 1988): 107-19.

18. R. Clarke et al., "Hyperhomocysteinemia: An independent risk factor for vascular disease," *New England Journal of Medicine* 324 (17) (25 April 1995): 1149-55.

19. B. Israelsson et al., "Homocysteine and myocardial infarction," *Atherosclerosis* 71 (1988): 227-33.

20. P. N. Hopkins et al., "Higher plasma homocyst[e]ine and increased susceptibility to adverse effects of low folate in early familial coronary artery disease," *Arteriosclerosis, Thrombosis, and Vascular Biology* 15 (September 1995): 1314-20.

21. D. G. Franken et al., "Treatment of mild hyperhomocysteinemia in vascular disease patients," *Arteriosclerosis & Thrombosis* 14 (3) (March 1994): 465-70.

22. B. M. Coull et al., "Elevated plasma homocyst[e]ine concentration as a possible independent risk factor for stroke," *Stroke* 21 (4) (April 1990): 572-76.

23. M. R. Malinow et al., "Prevalence of hyperhomocyst[e]inemia in patients with peripheral arterial occlusive disease," *Circulation* 79 (1989): 1180-88.

24. L. M. Taylor et al., "The association of elevated plasma homocyst[e]ine with progression of symptomatic peripheral arterial disease," *Journal of Vascular Surgery* 13 (1) (January 1991): 128-36.

25. S. S. Kang et al., "Intermediate hyperhomocysteinemia resulting from compound heterozygosity of methylenetetrahydrofolate reductase mutations," *American Journal of Human Genetics* 48 (3) (March 1991): 546-51.

26. See Note 1.

27. E. Arnesen et al., "Serum total homocysteine and coronary heart disease," *International Journal of Epidemiology* 24 (1955): 704-9.

28. H.I. Morrison et al., "Serum folate and risk of fatal coronary heart disease," *JAMA* 275 (1996); 1893-1896.

29. R. M. Russell, "A minimum of 13,500 deaths annually from coronary artery disease could be prevented by increasing folate intake to reduce homocysteine levels," *JAMA* 275 (1996): 1828-1829.

30. J. Selhub et al., "Association between plasma homocysteine concentrations and extracranial carotid-artery stenosis," *NEJM* 332 (2 February 1995): 286-91.

31. See Note 3.

32. S. S. Kang et al., "Homocysteinemia due to folate deficiency," *Metabolism* 36 (5) (May 1987): 458-62.

33. W. H. Giles et al., "Serum folate and risk of ischemic stroke: First National Health and Nutrition Examination Survey epidemiologic follow-up study," *Stroke* 26 (1995): 1166-70.

34. See Note 1.

35. L. E. Brattstrom et al., "Folic acid—an innocuous means to reduce plasma homocysteine," *Scandinavian Journal of Clinical Laboratory Investigations* 48 (1988): 215-21.

36. See Note 2.

37. G. Landgren et al., "Plasma homocysteine in acute myocardial infarction: homocysteine-lowering effect of folic acid," *Journal of Internal Medicine* 237 (April 1995): 381-88.

38. A. F. Subar et al., "Folate intake and food sources in the US population," *American Journal of Clinical Nutrition* 50 (September 1989): 508-16.

39. C. E. Butterworth et al., "Folic acid sfaety and toxicity: a brief review," *American Journal of Clinical Nutrition* 50 (August 1989): 353-58.

40. R. C. Campbell, "How safe are folic acid supplements?" *Archives of Internal Medicine* 156 (Aug 12/26, 1996): 1638:44

41. J. L. Mills et al., "Homocysteine metabolism in pregnancies complicated by neural tube defects," *Lancet* 345 (21 January 1995): 149-51.

42. P. N. Kirke et al., "Matrnal plasma folate and vitamin B12 are independent risk factors for neural tube defects," *Quarterly Journal of Medicine* 86 (November 1993): 703-8.

43. M. F. Fenech et al.,"Folate, vitamin B12, homocysteine status and chromosome damage rate in lymphocytes of older men," *Carcinogenesis* 18 (1997): 1329-36.

44. B. C. Blount et al.,"Folate deficiency causes uracil misincorporation into human DNA and chromosome breakage: implications for cancer and neuronal damage," Proceedings of the National Academy of Sciences of the USA 94 (April 1997): 3290-5.

45. C. Butterworth et al., "Folate deficiency and cervical dysplasia," *JAMA* 267 (1992): 528-33

46. C. Butterworth et al., "Oral folic acid supplementation for cervical dysplasia: a clinical intervention trial," American Journal of Obstetrical Gynecology 162 (1992): 803-9.

47. G. A. Paspatis et al., "Folate status and adenomatous colonic polyps," *Diseases of the Colon and Rectum* 38 (1955): 64-68.

48. R. S. Rivlin, speaking at The Health Benefits of Natural Phytoceuticals conference, Montreal, Canada, July 23, 1997

49. Y. I. Kim et al., "Folate deficiency in rats induces DNA strand breaks and hypomethylation within the p53 tumor suppressor gene," *American Journal of Clinical Nutrition* 65 (January 1997): 46-52.

50. M. Fava et al., "Folate, vitamin B12, and homocysteine in major depressive disorder," American Journal of Psychiatry 154 (March 1997): 426-8.

51. E. Joosten et al., "Is metabolic evidence for vitamin B-12 and folate deficiency more frequent in elderly patients with Alzheimer's disease?" *Journals of Gerontology Series A–Biological Sciences and Medical Sciences* 52 (1997): M76-M79.

52. B. C. Blount, op. cit.

53. M. Arnadottir et al., "The effect of high-dose pyridoxine and folic acid supplementation on serum lipid and plasma homocysteine concentrations in dialysis patients," *Clinical Nephrology* 40 (4) (October 1993): 236-40.

54. J. A. Friedman and J. T. Dwyer, "Hyperhomocysteinemia as a risk factor for cardiovascular disease in patients undergoing hemodialysis," *Nutrition Reviews* 53 (7) (1995): 197-201.

55. J. M. Ellis and K. S. McCully, "Prevention of myocardial infarction by vitamin B6," *Research Communications in Molecular Pathology and Pharmacology* 89 (August 1995): 208-220.

56. O. Nygard et al., "Plasma homocysteine levels and mortality in patients with coronary artery disease," *New England Journal of Medicine* 337 (July 24, 1997): 230-236.

57. M. van den Berg et al., "Hyperhomocysteinaemia and endothelial dysfunction in young patients with peripheral arterial occlusive disease," *European Journal of Clinical Investigation* 25 (3) (March 1995): 176-81.

58. H. J. Naurath et al., "Effects of vitamin B12, folate and vitamin B6 supplements in elderly people with normal serum vitamin concentrations," *Lancet* 346 (1995): 85-89.

59. See Note 2.

60. See Note 1.

61. P. J. Nestor and R. J. Stark, "Vitamin B12 myeloneuropathy precipitated by nitrous oxide anaesthesia," *Medical Journal of Australia* 165 (June 3, 1996): 174.

62. A. Araki et al., "Plasma homocysteine concentrations in Japanese patients with non-insulin-dependent diabetes mellitus: Effect of parenteral methylcobalamin treatment," *Atherosclerosis* 103 (November 1993): 149-57.

63. B. M. Cohen et al., "Brain choline uptake and cognitive function in middle age," *Biological Psychiatry* 41 (1997): 90S.

64. A. L. Stoll et al.,"Choline in the treatment of rapid-cycling bipolar disorder," *Biological Psychiatry* 40 (1996): 382-388.

65. C. Montero Brens et al., "Homocystinuria: Effectiveness of the treatment with pyridoxine, folic acid and betaine," *Anales Espan'oles de Pediatria* 39 (1) (July 1993): 37-41.

66. V. C. Wiley et al., "Free and protein-bound homocysteine and cysteine in cystathionine betasynthase deficiency: Interrelations during short- and long-term changes in plasma concentrations," *Metabolism: Clinical & Experimental* 38 (8) (August 1989): 734-39.

67. G. S. Tell et al., "Dietary fat intake and carotid artery wall thickness: the atherosclerosis risk in communities (ARIC) study," *American Journal of Epidemiology* 139 (1994): 979-89.
68. M. L. Burr and P. M. Sweetnam, "Vegetarianism, dietary fiber and mortality," *American Journal of Clinical Nutrition* 1982;36:873-7.
69. K. Resnicow et al., "Diet and serum lipids in vegan vegetarians: a model for risk reduction," *J Am Dietet Assoc* 1991;91:447-53.
70. D. Ornish et al., "Can lifestyle changes reverse coronary heart disease? The Lifestyle Heart Trial," *Lancet* 1990;336:129-33.
71. W. C. Willett et al., "Intake of trans fatty acids and risk of coronary heart disease among women," *Lancet* 1993;341:581-5.
72. J. W. Anderson and W. J. L. Chen, "Legumes and their soluble fiber: effect on cholesterol-rich lipoproteins.," In: Furda I, ed. Unconventional Sources of Dietary Fiber, Washington, DC, American Chemical Society, 1983.
73. C. M. Ripsin et al., "Oat products and lipid lowering—a meta-analysis," *JAMA* 1992;267:3317-25.
74. B. Halliwell, "Oxidation of low-density lipoproteins: Questions of initiation, propagation, and the effect of antioxidants," *Am J Clin Nutr* 61:670S-677S, 1995.
75. J. Regnstrom, "Susceptibility to low-density lipoprotein oxidation and coronary atherosclerosis in man," *Lancet* 339:1183-1186, 1992.
76. J. Price and F. Fowkes, "Antioxidant vitamins in the prevention of cardiovascular disease," *Eur Heart J* 18:719-727, 1997.
77. E. B. Rimm et al., "Vitamin E consumption and the risk of coronary heart disease in men," *New England Journal of Medicine* 328 (20) (1993): 1450-1456.
78. M. Stampfer et al., "Vitamin E consumption and the risk of coronary disease in women," *New Engl J Med* 328:1444-1449, 1993.
79. N. Stephens et al., "Randomised controlled trial of vitamin E in patients with coronary disease: Cambridge Heart Antioxidant Study (CHAOS)," *Lancet* 347:781-786, 1996.
80. J. Simon, "Vitamin C & heart disease," *Nutrition Report* 10 (1992): 57, 64.
81 S. Keli et al., "Dietary flavonoids, antioxidant vitamins, and incidence of stroke," *Arch Intern Med* 154:637-642, 1996.
82. D. Siscovick et al., "Dietary intake and cell membrane levels of long-chain n-3 polyunsaturated fatty acids and the risk of primary cardiac arrest," *JAMA* 274:1363-1367, 1996.
83 M. Steiner et al., "A double-blind crossover study in moderately hypercholesterolemic men that compared the effect of aged garlic extract and placebo administration on blood lipids," *American Journal of Clinical Nutrition*, 64(6):866-870, December 1996.
84. J. Anderson et al., "Meta-analysis of the effects of soy protein intake on serum lipids," *New Engl J Med* 333:276-282, 1995.
85. S. Khosla et al., "Cardiovascular effects of nicotine: relation to deleterious effects of cigarette smoking," *Am Heart J* 1994;127:1669-71.
86. I. Kawachi et al., "Smoking cessation and time course of decreased risks of coronary heart disease in middle-aged women," *Archives of Internal Medicine* 154 (1994):169-175.

87. J. Pekkanen et al., "Reduction of premature mortality by high physical activity: a 20-year follow-up of middle-aged Finnish men," *Lancet* 1987;1:1473-7.
88. J. J. Duncan et al., "Women walking for health and fitness—how much is enough?" *JAMA* 1991;266:3295-99.
89. H. B. Hubert et al., "Obesity as an independent risk factor for cardiovascular disease: a 26-year follow-up of participants in the Framingham Heart Study," *Circulation* 1983;67:968-77.
90. R. R. Wing and R. W. Jeffery, "Effect of modest weight loss on changes in cardiovascular risk factors," *International Journal of Obesity* 19 (1995): 67-73.
91. I. Kawachi et al., "A prospective study of anger and coronary heart disease," *Circulation* 1996;94:2090-5.
92. W. Jiang et al., "Mental stress-induced myocardial ischemia and cardiac events," *JAMA* 1996;275:1651-6.
93. M. Friedman et al., "Alteration of type A behavior and reduction in cardiac recurrences in postmyocardial infarction patients," *Am Heart J* 1984;108:237-48.